MAKE-UP
Manual

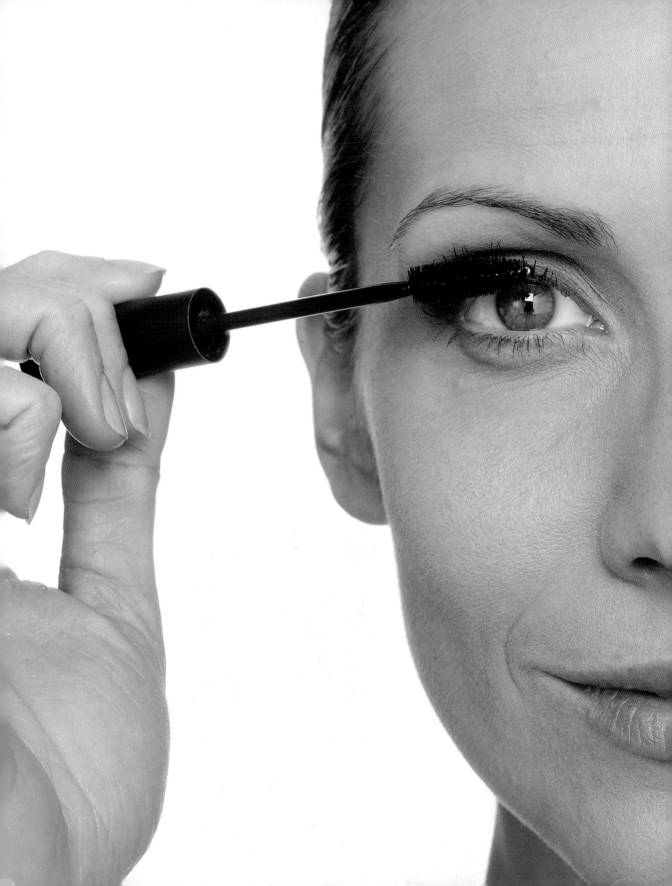

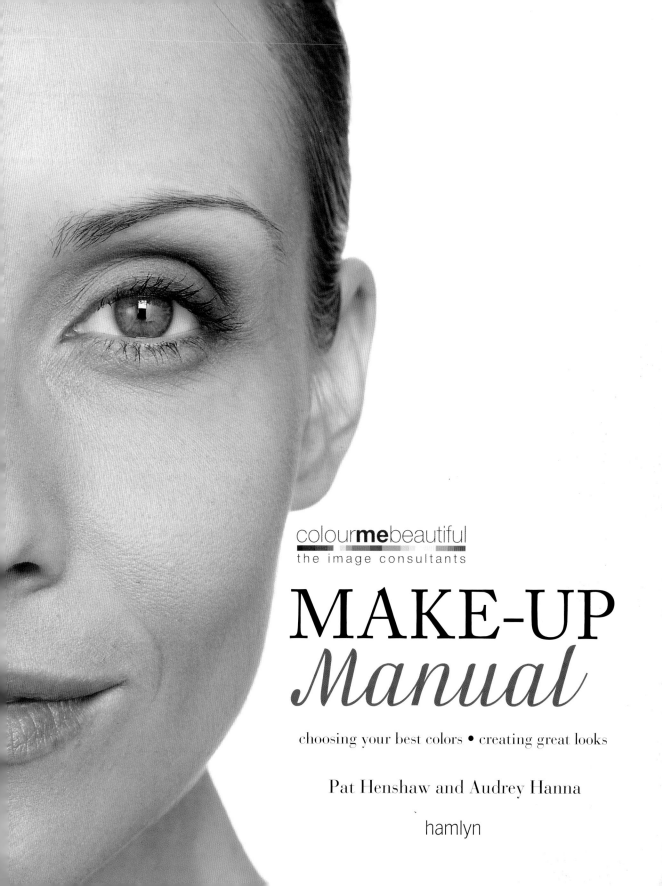

colourme**beautiful**
the image consultants

MAKE-UP
Manual

choosing your best colors • creating great looks

Pat Henshaw and Audrey Hanna

hamlyn

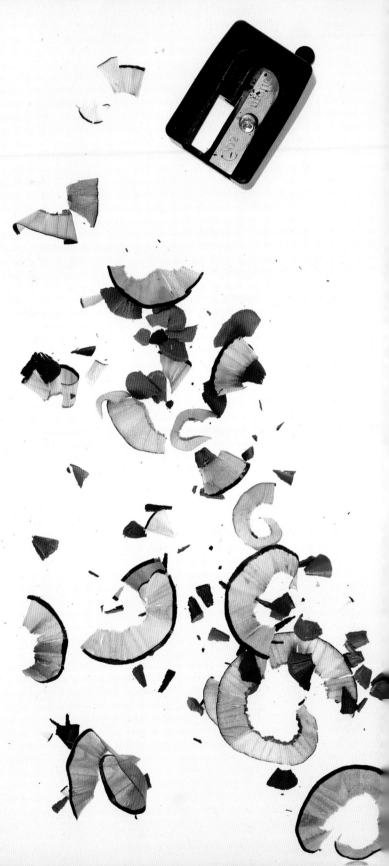

An Hachette UK Company
www.hachette.co.uk

First published in Great Britain in 2012 by Hamlyn,
a division of Octopus Publishing Group Ltd
Endeavour House
189 Shaftesbury Avenue
London
WC2H 8JY
www.octopusbooksusa.com

Distributed in the US by
Hachette Book Group USA
237 Park Avenue
New York NY 10017 USA

Distributed in Canada by
Canadian Manda Group
165 Dufferin Street
Toronto, Ontario, Canada M6K 3H6

ISBN 978-0-600-62331-1

Printed and bound in China

10 9 8 7 6 5 4 3 2 1

Every effort has been made to reproduce the
colors in this book accurately; however, the
printing process can lead to some discrepancies.
The color samples provided should be used as
a guideline only.

CONTENTS

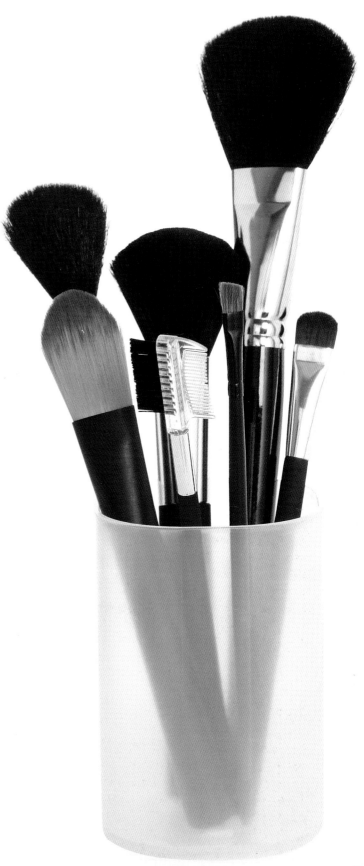

INTRODUCTION

For close to 30 years, Colour Me Beautiful have been the leading experts in the field of color analysis and styling. Our worldwide team of highly trained and motivated consultants has groomed, cajoled, and inspired women of all ages and from all walks of life to embrace color into their lives. The greatest impact color has is with make-up.

HOW TO USE THIS BOOK

To make the most of your make-up and create a look that complements your style, your age, and the occasion, it is essential to understand your skin, and get to know your personal coloring. This book offers many tips and loads of advice to help you, from identifying your skin type and establishing a skincare routine, to the type and colors of make-up that will suit you and the most flattering ways to apply it.

Your skin is your face's canvas. The first chapter looks at the importance of understanding your skin's needs, from what we put inside ourselves to establishing a skincare routine. It gives advice on how to prevent and disguise the signs of aging as well as how to project healthy, glowing skin. Skincare has made massive advances in the last decade, so don't skip it even if you have good skin.

The next chapter guides you through the vast choice available at the make-up counter, from foundations and powders to mascaras and eye liners, with helpful advice on the range of options, what tools you need to apply them, and how to apply them to create different make-up looks. Once you understand application techniques, the next step is to discover your coloring type, which will lead you to finding the shades of make-up that work for you. With a palette of colors to choose from for each coloring type, we'll show you how to apply them to create different looks that will enhance, flatter, hide, and rejuvenate.

With so many options available, it can be difficult to know how much, or how little, make-up to apply. Chapter Four shows you how to build on a basic look from "barely there" to a full-blown "night glamour" makeover, with suggestions for each coloring type. As with your wardrobe, it is important that your make-up is appropriate for the different stages in your life. You'll find plenty of tips and advice on looking good and making the most of your make-up through the years.

Throughout the book you'll find tricks of the trade, such as how to make your eyes look bigger or your mouth look smaller, along with special tips on how to flatter your face shape. The final chapter guides you through the finishing touches that will complete the perfect look.

COLOR ME BEAUTIFUL

Thousands of our clients' lives have been changed by following our simple guidelines and advice based on our color analysis system, from coordinating their wardrobes to developing a positive attitude to their personal appearance.

The Colour Me Beautiful color analysis system allows us to focus on a basis of six dominant coloring types: Light, Deep, Warm, Cool, Clear, and Soft, which are used in this book. Within each group there will, of course, be many variations depending on eye color, skin tone, and hair shade. Follow the general guidelines given in the book to help assess how to wear the recommended shades of eye shadows, blushes, eye pencils, lip pencils, and lipsticks—how and where you apply make-up is as important as the shade or color in creating a successful look.

OUR MAKE-UP RANGE

Most cosmetic manufacturers follow fashion trends rather than looking at what tones, shades, and colors will suit different people. In 1988, Colour Me Beautiful launched its own range of cosmetics, looking at the best colors for each coloring type, thus enhancing the client's look rather than distracting from it.

Not only have we developed a range of colors that we know work with our typical coloring types, but we regularly review new fashion shades to stay current. The colors mentioned in this book are guidelines—we have used names that reflect the shades and will help you identify similar tones at the cosmetics counter.

BELOW Although our gorgeous model below has perfect skin, she does look a bit tired without any make-up on.

BELOW Well-applied make-up can make you look more alive, healthier, and younger.

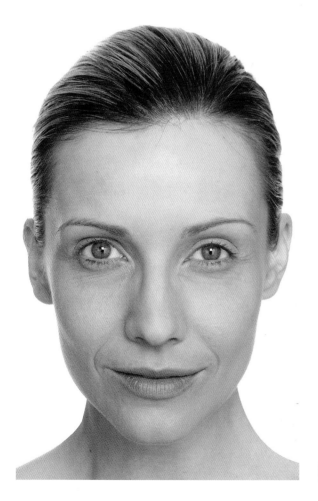
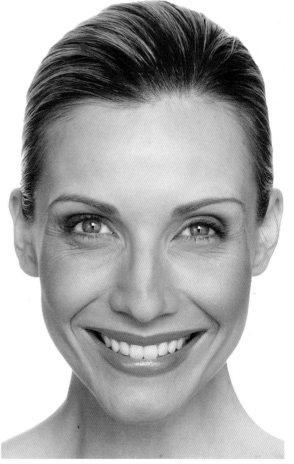

SKINCARE

"Beauty is only skin deep," but so often we forget that beautiful skin is achieved through care and effort, not just luck. Yes, genes do play a part in how our skin looks, but with modern products and a healthy lifestyle, we can all improve the canvas that we apply our make-up to. Understanding how to care for your skin, from identifying your skin type to choosing the right products for you, is the first step to flawless make-up.

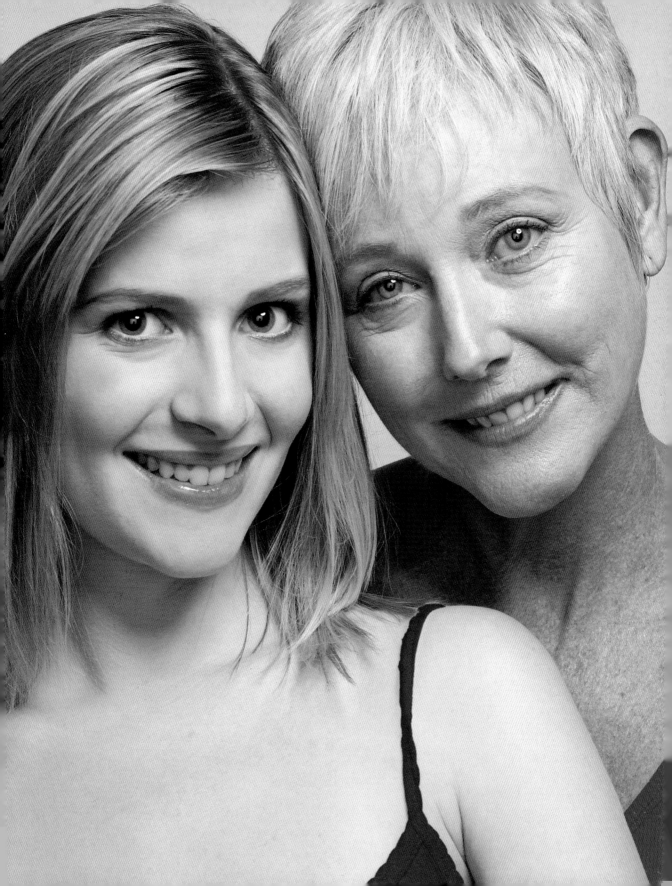

CARING FOR YOUR SKIN

The skin is the largest organ we have and one of the most accessible—we can see it and feel it. Your face, in particular, is a mirror of your well-being. Take a moment to get to know your skin and the best ways of maintaining its youthful appearance, from the inside out. Once your skin is at its optimum health, your make-up will serve to enhance and build on that inner beauty.

THE SKIN'S STRUCTURE

Your skin is constantly working to keep bacteria and toxins out while keeping every other part in. To better understand your skin's behavior, we need to first understand what it is made up of. The skin consists of three layers: the epidermis, the dermis, and the hypodermis (subcutaneous layer). The thickness of the skin varies in different parts of the body—   it is thinnest around the eyes (especially the eyelids) and thicker in the areas subjected to most wear and tear, such as the soles of the feet and, to a lesser extent, the hands.

EPIDERMIS

This is the top layer of the skin, which is about as thin as a sheet of paper. This is the outer "superficial" layer, which we can see and which acts as our body's shield against the outside world. The whole process of skincare is to keep the epidermis healthy and plump, as this will protect the the dermis, which is where aging signs appear.

The acid mantle is a thin oily film that sits on the surface of the skin and acts as a barrier to bacteria, viruses, and other potential contaminants that might penetrate the skin. For most people, the pH (potential hydrogen) content of the acid mantle is about 4.5 to 5.5—it is this slight acidity that neutralizes any harmful contaminants. Maintaining the skin pH at the proper level is vital to protecting ourselves from harmful bacteria, which can lead to acne, infection, or irritation. Use skincare products with pH balancing factors that are specifically designed for your skin type.

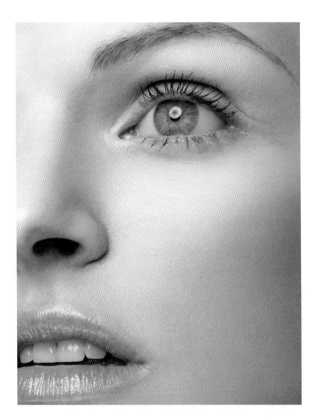

ABOVE Taking care of your skin through a good diet and proper skincare routine will give you an overall healthy appearance.

The skin's outer layer works in a very similar way to an escalator. On the "bottom step" are fresh new cells, which constantly work their way upward. When the cells reach the skin's surface they begin to die, forming the protective layer of dead cells that we see.

The epidermis is the part of your skin that skincare products have been designed to work on. When we are young, this layer replaces itself every 16 days or so, giving us fresh, healthy-looking skin. As we age, this renewal process slows down, and by the time we hit 35 the outer layer only replaces itself about once a month, causing our skin to lose its youthful appearance.

A good skincare routine and balanced diet will help keep the acid mantle balanced.

DERMIS

This is the underlying layer of the epidermis, which acts as the skin's support, composed of elastic tissue known as collagen. Through this framework runs a network of nerves and blood vessels. In young, healthy skin, collagen is arranged in parallel bundles that lie alongside each other and have the ability to stretch and then resume their original shape. They give young skin its suppleness, smoothness, and plumpness. As we age, the integrity of the collagen bundles is lost and the fibers split; the bundles begin to break up and the parallel arrangements disintegrate, causing the skin to sag, wrinkle, and become thinner. Unlike the epidermis, the dermis does not replenish and is a permanent layer.

The dermis provides nourishment for the epidermis through blood vessels that transport oxygen, water, and nutrients. It also contains sebaceous glands, adjoining the hair follicle. The glands resemble a bunch of grapes and produce a natural oil called sebum. It's the sebum that lubricates the skin to make it more pliable and flexible. It also prevents dryness and cracking. These secretions, in conjunction with the sweat deposits, also form the acid mantle. The dermis also contains:

- **Sweat glands** to excrete waste products and water. Sweat is the body's way of cooling down. While doing so it pumps moisture onto the outer layer of the skin that combines with dead skin cells, sebum oils, and waste products—all of which need to be removed.

- **Lymphatic vessels** to remove waste products and flush the system.

- **Muscle and nerve fibers** to warn the body of outside stimuli.

- **Oil glands** to provide lubrication—overproduction during puberty can cause skin problems; as we age, these glands slow down, causing dryness.

UVA and UVB rays can break down the dermis: use a moisturizer and sunscreens with SPF 30 or higher.

HYPODERMIS

The third and bottom layer is the hypodermis, also known as the subcutaneous layer. It is mostly fat and its main function is to provide insulation and regulate body temperature. It helps conserve heat in the winter and give off heat in the summer, and it supports and gives contour and firmness to your shape. To keep it healthy, drink plenty of water and avoid yo-yo dieting, which can deprive you of essential nutrients.

HUMAN SKIN

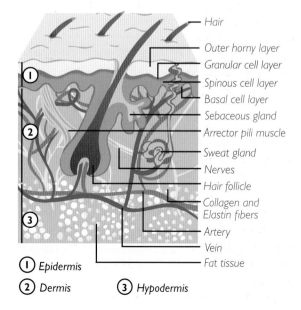

Hair
Outer horny layer
Granular cell layer
Spinous cell layer
Basal cell layer
Sebaceous gland
Arrector pili muscle
Sweat gland
Nerves
Hair follicle
Collagen and Elastin fibers
Artery
Vein
Fat tissue

① Epidermis
② Dermis
③ Hypodermis

HEALTHY LIFESTYLE FOR SKIN

Without a doubt, a proper skincare routine and good-quality skincare products will provide noticeable effects for your skin. However, it's also important to remember to feed your skin from the inside—that's where beautiful skin starts. Only with the winning combination of a healthy lifestyle and great skincare can you expect to get the best results for your skin.

HEALTHY DIET

Go for food that is fresh and unprocessed. Processed foods are full of additives that remove the nutrients that our skin desperately needs. Eat the correct balance of foods and you'll feed your skin the vital nutrients to help it stay soft, supple and blemish-free.

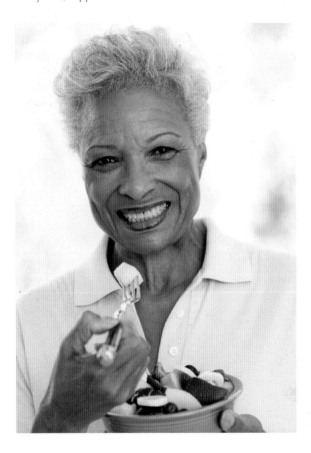

- Fruit and vegetables contain powerful antioxidants that help protect the skin against damage from cigarette smoke, pollution, and the sun's UV rays. Vitamin C is one of the most powerful antioxidants and is found in all fruit and vegetables, but is especially high in blackcurrants, blueberries, broccoli, guava, kiwi fruits, oranges, papaya, strawberries, and red peppers.

- Eating foods that contain sulfur can help keep skin smooth—garlic and onions are full of it.

- Good fats or unsaturated fats. We need some fat in our diet because it helps the body absorb certain nutrients. Good fats can be found in avocados, nuts, and seeds—they provide essential fatty acids, which act as a natural moisturizer for your skin, keeping it supple because of the healthy dose of vitamin E. Omega oils are an excellent source of fatty acids and can be found in oily fish such as salmon and mackerel.

- Zinc-rich foods, such as wheat germ, liver, pumpkin seeds, sardines, and oysters, help repair skin damage and keep it soft and supple.

- Foods rich in vitamin A help new skin cells to grow. Liver, eggs, milk, and oily fish are good sources.

Don't expect an overnight miracle once you start to make changes to your diet. It can take from a month to six weeks to see or feel the visible effects.

LEFT **Having a balanced diet not only makes you feel better on the inside but gives your skin a healthy, glowing appearance.**

WELL HYDRATED

Even mild dehydration will cause your skin to look dry, tired, and slightly grey. Drink plenty of water to rehydrate your skin and to eliminate toxins from the body: aim for eight glasses a day (about 1 to 2 quarts). Coffee, tea, and juices do count, but for really great skin stick to plain water. If you work in an air-conditioned environment, keep a large bottle of water on your desk to remind you to drink. Even drying your hair or driving with the heater on may dry your skin out.

REST AND RELAXATION

One of the first places that lack of sleep shows is on your face, with dark circles or puffiness under the eyes. Try if you can to get 7 to 8 hours of sleep each night. Not only will you feel refreshed, but being well rested can also relieve stress—another factor that can cause skin problems, including early aging, eczema, pimples, and dry skin.

EXERCISE

We all know that exercise improves your health, but it also has the added benefit of showcasing that health through your skin with a rosy, healthy-looking glow. Exercise helps unclog pores and flush out toxins from our skin. If you exercise outdoors, try to do so in the morning or early evening, avoiding the middle of the day when UV rays are at the highest. Regardless of what time, remember to wear a moisturizer and an SPF sunscreen to protect your skin.

Remove any make-up before you exercise, otherwise it can lead to clogged pores, which cause blackheads. After your workout, wash your hands immediately and change out of sweaty clothes and shower as soon as possible—the evaporated sweat may leave behind salt that will clog up your pores again. Drink plenty of liquids, too, to replenish those that you've lost through perspiration.

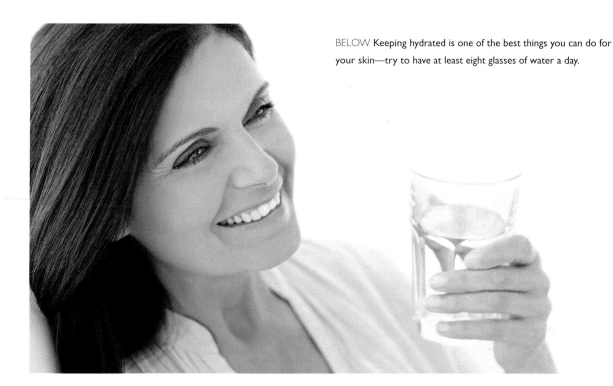

BELOW **Keeping hydrated is one of the best things you can do for your skin—try to have at least eight glasses of water a day.**

IDENTIFYING YOUR SKIN TYPE

Before you think about make-up, it's important that your skin is as clear and healthy as possible. Good skincare is about identifying your skin's tendencies and characteristics so that you can treat it accordingly. Whether your skin is normal, dry, oily, sensitive, or combination, you can encourage it to its full potential by following a proper skincare routine every day.

Most of us know how our skin feels, so identifying your skin type should be fairly easy. Keep in mind, though, once you start using a good skincare routine, your skin type may change.

NORMAL SKIN

This type of skin is smooth in texture and evenly toned with no enlarged pores, rarely suffers from breakouts and

BELOW **No matter what your skin type, be sure to follow a skincare routine both in the morning and at night.**

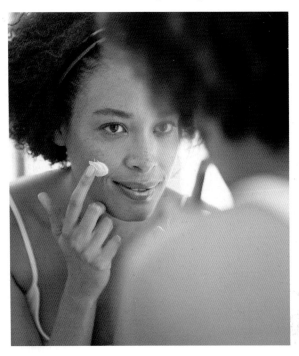

often feels soft and velvety. You are truly blessed if you have this type of skin—smooth and unblemished. Every care needs to be taken to ensure that this wonderful skin lasts over time.

DRY SKIN

This skin type is often aggravated by being overexposed to harsh elements—wind, sun, cold air, and even indoor heating and air conditioning. The skin may appear flaky and/or feel rough to the touch. Generally, wrinkles develop early and dryness tends to intensify with age —proper skincare can help alleviate this. The plus side is that pores are almost invisible, making the skin less susceptible to breakouts.

OILY SKIN

This skin type often feels greasy, even after cleansing, and has visible open pores, which makes it prone to breakouts and blackheads. To keep the pores from clogging, oily skin needs special cleansing. The good news is that it will develop fewer wrinkles over time and maintains its elasticity longer.

COMBINATION SKIN

This skin type combines both oily and dry areas. It is oily in the T-zone—across the forehead and down the nose and chin, where most oil glands are found—but drier in the cheeks. The skincare routine needs to absorb the oil in the T-zone and also moisturize the cheeks, so a mixture of skincare routines is required.

SENSITIVE SKIN

This type of skin can be oily and/or dry and can feel itchy, bumpy, or flaky. There are many factors that can cause sensitive skin, including stress, extreme changes in weather, hormonal changes that come with age, dyes and fragrances in cosmetics and skincare products, poor diet, dehydration, allergens, and heavy pollution. There are many skincare products designed for sensitive skin, from those that are fragrance-free to those with natural ingredients. If you experience major recurring symptoms, consider seeing a dermatologist —you may have an underlying skin condition such as dermatitis, eczema, psoriasis, or ichthyosis. Many of these skin conditions are treatable, if not manageable, and can be helped with medication.

CHANGING NEEDS

Your skin type may change over time, from seasonal change to more long-term change as you age. Adapt your skincare routine accordingly. Young skins tend to be more oily and mature skins drier. Stress, climate, and medications can also affect the surface of the skin.

SKINCARE TIP

Never change your entire skincare regime all at once, in case of a reaction. Introduce products one by one to establish which ones suit you.

BELOW Sometimes a bit of trial and error with different products will be required before you discover your perfect skincare.

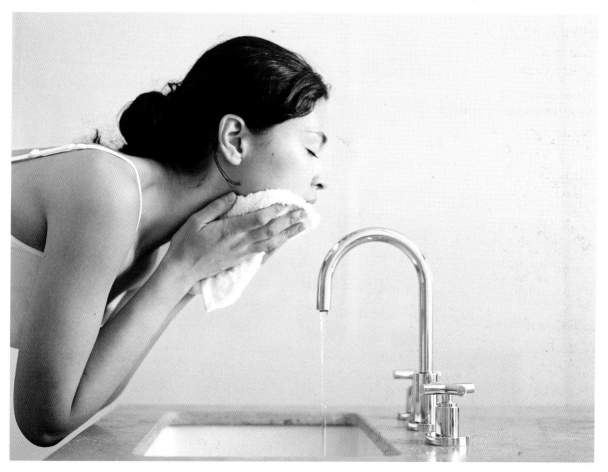

SKINCARE ROUTINES

A good skincare routine is an insurance policy for later life—the earlier you start, the longer you will have healthy-looking skin. Be aware of any changes to your skin type, especially the effects of the weather, and adapt your routine or products accordingly. Even if you are busy, don't skip a step. Once your routine becomes a habit, you can enjoy healthy, glowing skin for years to come.

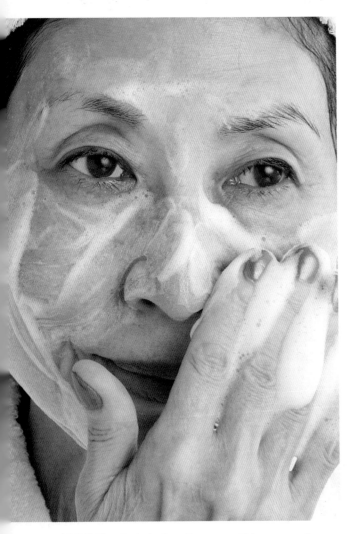

ABOVE **Cleansing is the first skincare step. Make sure you choose a cleanser that is best for your skin type.**

WHAT IS PROPER SKINCARE?

There are three daily skincare steps that everyone should follow, no matter what your skin type, both in the morning and at night: cleanse, tone, and moisturize.

STEP 1: CLEANSE

You need to cleanse to remove excess oil, grime, make-up, waste products eliminated from the skin, and dead skin cells, which can all clog pores. It is much more than just getting rid of dirt, which is what soap does. (Soap also leaves deposits on the skin that can clog and dry the skin more.) Instead, you need to get deep inside the pores, which only a proper cleanser can do.

Overnight the skin expels impurities, perspiration, and excess oils onto its surface, so it's important that they are removed before applying your make-up in the morning. Start by cleansing, follow by toning, and finish with a moisturizer. At night, before you apply your cleanser, use a gentle eye make-up remover on a damp cotton pad. Start downward on the top of the lid, then work from the outer edge of the eye inward to avoid stretching the delicate skin. Eye make-up removers are specifically designed to dissolve and remove mascara, eye pencils, and eye shadows.

There are several types of cleanser:

- **Foam or gel cleansers for oily, normal, and combination skin:** Normally applied to the face with your hands and rinsed off with water. Particularly good if you like the feel of washing your face.

- **Lotion cleansers for normal and combination skins:** Gently rub into the face with your fingertips and remove with your toner applied on a damp cotton pad. Some lotion cleansers can be rinsed off with water, but be sure that no cleanser is left on your face, because this can cause blemishes.

- **Cream cleansers for dry and sensitive skins:** Gently massage onto your face with your fingertips, then remove with your toner applied on a damp cotton pad. Keep using damp cotton pads until no more make-up appears on the pad. Try not to use water when cleansing, especially if you live in a hard-water area, because this will leave the skin feeling taut and dry from the minerals in the water.

- **Facial wipes:** Handy for traveling because they are quick and easy to use, but should not be used on a regular basis as they don't cleanse as deeply as a cleanser, and tend to be harsh on the skin.

STEP 2: TONE

You need to tone to tighten pores, refine, and rejuvenate. No matter what your skin type, avoid an alcohol-based toner, as alcohol is very harsh and strips the skin of its natural oils, which keep the skin nourished. Instead, look for toners with healing or antibacterial ingredients, such as witch hazel or chamomile.

There are two types of toner:

- **Alcohol-free toners:** Good for oily, normal, and combination skins. Apply on damp cotton pads to dissolve and remove cleanser.

- **Skin fresheners or natural toners**, such as rosewater or orange flower water, are great for dry and sensitive skins. These have gentle stimulating properties that improve the skin's circulation.

STEP 3: MOISTURIZE

You need to moisturize to hydrate, revive the skin, and keep it supple. Everyone needs moisturizer, even those with oily skin, as it helps all skin types retain moisture.

Most daytime moisturizers contain vitamins, natural oils (such as avocado), and sun filters to protect the skin. After cleansing and toning, apply moisturizer in the morning and night cream in the evening to damp skin to help counteract evaporation. Apply with your fingertips, gently massaging over the whole face, avoiding the eye area—too much moisturizer can make them puffy.

Moisturizer also forms a protective layer on the skin when applied before make-up, preventing the make-up

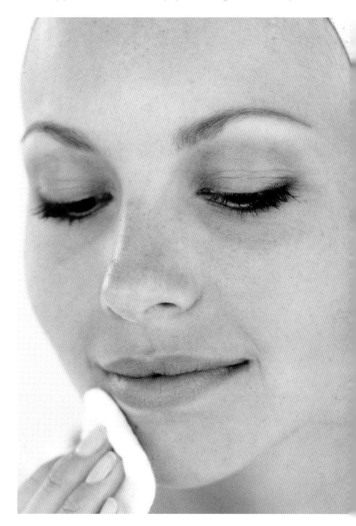

ABOVE **Using a toner will guarantee perfectly clean skin, as it removes the final traces of your cleanser as well as any excess oils.**

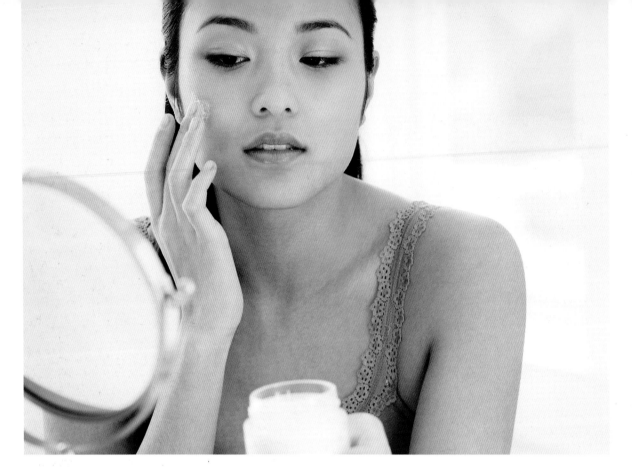

from being absorbed into the pores and helping it to go on smoothly and evenly.

There are several types of moisturizer:

- **Liquid or lightweight moisturizers:** Ideal for normal and oily skins. It may sound counterintuitive for those with oily skins to use moisturizers—keep in mind, though, that they do not add water but contain humectants, which keep the skin's natural moisture in and prevent oil glands from becoming overactive.

- **Cream moisturizers:** Ideal for dry or sensitive skins. If you have combination skin, you may feel you want to use two types of moisturizer—a light one for the T-zone and a heavier cream for the dry areas.

- **Eye products:** It's important to use products that are designed for the eye area, used sparingly, rather than face creams, which are too rich and heavy and will result in puffy eyes. For all skin types, eye gels are good for puffy eyes and dark circles. They are normally applied in the morning around the eye area

ABOVE **Moisturizing and nourishing is your insurance against a dry and aging skin.**

before the application of eye make-up, to keep the skin nourished during the day. Eye creams are applied at night with gentle tapping motions, to nourish and help prevent fine lines and crêpiness.

- **Night creams:** All skin types, including oily skin, will benefit from the use of a night cream, which will

SKINCARE TIPS

- Think seasonally—you may need a lighter moisturizer in the summer when your skin gets a little oilier, or a richer, creamier prouct in winter when the cold can cause dryness.

- Remember to always treat your neck as well as your face, otherwise you'll end up with a lovely face and a wrinkly, crêpey neck.

penetrate the outer layer of the skin, have a plumping effect on the dehydrated skin cells, and are designed to slow down the production of the skin's natural oil.

OTHER PRODUCTS

- **Exfoliators:** Designed to remove the dead skin cells from the surface of the skin, revealing the new and plumper cells beneath. They may be used as often as you feel necessary, depending on your skin type and age—2 to 3 times a week is generally sufficient. Avoid facial scrubs that contain nut kernels, which are designed for parts of the body where the skin is thicker such as hands and soles of the feet.

- **Serums and rejuvenating lotions:** Most contain agents to counteract free radicals in the atmosphere.

BELOW Not only a great pampering treat, the regular use of a clay mask can reduce the appearance of blackheads.

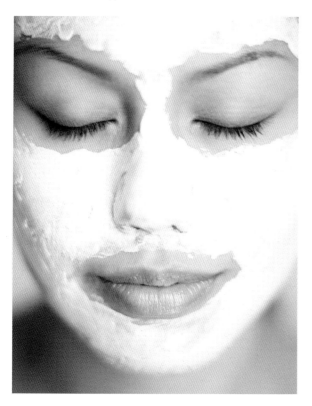

They improve the appearance of the skin by plumping up the skin cells in the epidermis and encouraging the cell renewal process. They vary tremendously in price, and the most expensive are not necessarily the most effective. Find one to suit your skin type and budget.

- **Face masks:** Help to exfoliate by removing dead skin cells. They also stimulate blood circulation and lymphatic drainage, which help take impurities away from the skin, thereby encouraging oily skin to become less oily and dry skin to become less dry. It's important to use the right type of mask for your skin type:

- **Clay or hard-setting masks:** Great for oily skins and enlarged pores. The clay forms a seal over the pores, causing the skin to move debris up to the surface and the pores to tighten. These masks work best applied immediately after steaming the face: fill a bowl with hot water and sit with your face over the bowl and a towel over your head. Be prepared for blemishes to appear after using these masks; however, after a few days you'll have a radiant glow. Regular use of masks will keep blemishes at bay.

- **Gel masks and soft masks:** A relaxing treatment for dry and more mature skins. They hydrate and firm rather than tighten. Gel masks stay soft on the skin throughout the treatment.

SKINCARE TIP

To avoid frequently buying new lotions, such as your eye make-up remover or toner, you can prolong their use by applying them with a damp cotton pad instead of applying directly onto a dry pad, which absorbs more liquid. This also ensures that the fine fibers of the pad do not come away on your face.

COMMON ISSUES

At any time during your life you may experience minor problems with your skin. These are often caused by hormonal changes, medications, diet, stress, and even poor health. Most of these conditions are temporary and can be treated at home—if they persist, however, seek advice from your beautician or in extreme cases, your doctor or a dermatologist.

BLACKHEADS

A blackhead is a plug of sebum that is trapped in the sebaceous gland duct and oxidizes on contact with the air, turning it black.

Avoid: Products that contain Isopropyl myristate, a synthetic oil often used in cheap skincare products as an emollient. It can irritate the skin, aggravate blackheads, and block pores.

Treatment: Thorough cleansing, exfoliating, and skin brushing are good for prevention and removal. If you are prone to blackheads, regular clay face masks can also help. In severe cases a hydradermie treatment (see page 22) may be required. Never attempt to squeeze or remove blackheads with your fingertips. The skin is so fine that you can easily cause an infection.

MILIA (OR WHITEHEADS)

These are tiny pearly white (or sometimes pale yellow) bumps that appear under the surface of the skin. They are often found around the eyes, nose, and along the cheekbones. They're a type of cyst filled with a substance called keratin, a protein that gives strength to the skin. It is not fully understood why they appear and why some people get them while others don't. It can be hereditary, and they can also be aggravated by using heavy creams, make-up, or other products that contain mineral oil and wax.

Avoid: Heavy creams and make-up. Also avoid picking and squeezing at them, which can lead to scarring.

Treatment: Facial exfoliating should keep milia at bay. It removes the top layer of skin, which can enable the cysts to fall out. A simple facial sauna will help remove dead skin cells and debris from the skin, too. Professional facial treatment is an option (see page 22).

BELOW A facial brush is a great way to exfoliate and loosen dead skin cells, which helps keep the skin clear.

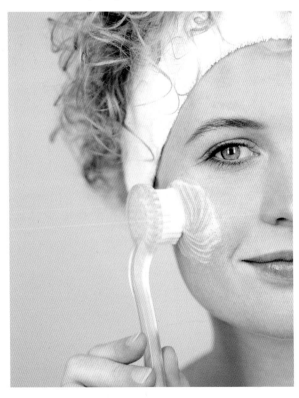

OPEN PORES

Open or enlarged pores are ones that are visible on the surface of the skin. They can attract waste products, dirt, and grime, which can all get trapped.

Avoid: For oily and young skins, avoid skin-stripping products, such as facial wipes. These only result in an overproduction of sebum, which can cause open pores.

For older skin, avoid heavy products that contain lanolin, and always tone after cleansing. Otherwise, the muscles around the pores become stretched and open pores will appear.

Treatment: Good cleansing, toning, and exfoliating are key. Try using face masks—either clay or gel—regularly, to stimulate the skin.

ACNE

A few spots or blemishes that appear monthly are not considered acne. Acne is a clinical condition where the skin is infected; it is characterized by scaly red skin, blackheads and whiteheads, pimples, and possible scarring. It is often caused by the overproduction of testosterone.

Avoid: Very rich skincare products and stripping products, such as alcohol-based cleansers, which will only cause the skin to produce more oils.

Treatment: Good skin hygiene is essential to keep acne under control. Look for products that are designed for oily skin (but not oil-stripping ones) that reduce the overproduction of sebum. In severe cases, medical advice should be sought. Foundation sponges, make-up brushes, and washcloths are a haven for bacteria, so they must be washed regularly to avoid reinfection. Also, try to stop touching your face with your hands, which may transport bacteria.

ROSACEA

Often distinguished by a red, flushed appearance around the nose and cheeks, rosacea tends to be more

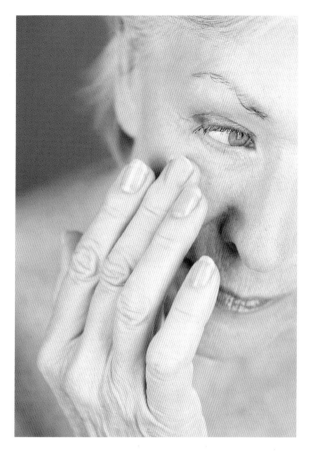

ABOVE **If you suffer from rosacea, use very gentle movements on your face when applying products—too much pressure will only increase the redness.**

common in older women and can be food, stress or temperature related.

Avoid: Most sufferers will know what triggers their rosacea breakouts, for example, coffee, wine, cheese, or spicy foods. Skincare products containing fragrances, alcohol, and fruit acids can also be triggers for rosacea, so they are best avoided.

Treatment: Use calming products, such as chamomile, rather than stimulating products with an alcohol base. Skin primers with a green base are great at hiding a breakout. Drinking plenty of water can also calm down the redness.

PROFESSIONAL TREATMENTS

Preventive measures, such as a good skincare routine, is always the best way to slow down the aging process and keep your skin glowing and healthy. Treatments are often very relaxing and help maintain good skin for the future. Once aging signs occur, there are treatments that can disguise fine lines, wrinkles, and sagging skin without resorting to invasive facial surgery.

Before making an appointment for one of the treatments listed below, check out your practitioner or beautician's certifications and qualifications.

FACIALS

A facial can be any beauty treatment for your face. Those performed by professional beauticians in a salon or spa fall into two main categories:

MANUAL, HAND HOLISTIC FACIALS

These use natural products, such as aromatherapy oils, which help lymphatic drainage and improve the condition of the skin. Most facial treatments will include cleansing, exfoliation, massage, and a mask appropriate for your skin type. This type of facial stimulates circulation, drains the lymphatic system, and relaxes the client, which is probably one of the most important benefits of this type of treatment. Treatments need to be repeated on a regular basis to maintain effectiveness.

TECHNICAL FACIALS

A Microdermabrasion machine uses aluminum oxide crystals to gently exfoliate the upper layers of the skin while gently sucking the crystals and dead skin debris back into the machine, removing blackheads and other impurities. Once these dead skin cells are removed, newer, more vibrant skin is revealed, making your skin feel and look smoother, healthier, and more youthful.

Hydradermie uses customized fortified gels designed to resolve any issues with your skin. Using precision massaging movements, the Hydraderm machine rollers use mild electrotherapy to help the active ingredients in the gel penetrate deep into the skin to remove impurities and toxins. The skin is then more receptive to targeted ingredients such as deep cleansing or moisturizing. Ideally, this treatment needs to be repeated on a monthly basis to maintain the results.

CHEMICAL SKIN PEELS

Skin peels are chemical masks that often contain Alpha Hydroxy Acids (AHAs), used to smooth the texture of the skin. The AHAs stimulate the skin to excrete dead and damaged skin cells, thereby quickly bringing new, plumper cells to the surface. Chemical peels can be varied according to how deep you want the peel. Superficial wrinkles and pigmentation issues can be improved by superficial peels. Deeper wrinkles require deeper peels. Care must be taken not to repeat the peel too often, as they can lead to the skin being sensitized. Great care must be taken afterward when exposing the skin to sunlight. A chemical peel should only be conducted by a professional beautician or dermatologist.

BOTOX AND SKIN FILLERS

Botox is a substance that is injected into the dermal layer of the skin through a fine needle, which relaxes the contractions of the muscles by blocking the nerve impulses. The result is that muscles can no longer contract, so wrinkles relax and soften. It usually takes 2 to 4 days to see the cosmetic improvement, and the effects generally last for 4 to 6 months.

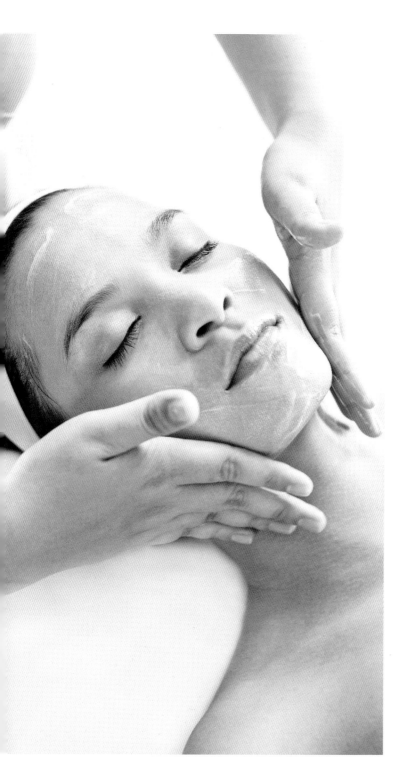

This is an invasive procedure and should be administered by a licensed professional, preferably a medical practitioner.

HAIR REMOVAL

There are various types of facial hair removal, some that can be done at home and some that need to be administered by a professional:

- **Tweezing:** Best for small areas such as eyebrows (see pages 118–119).

- **Bleaching:** Best for fine, downy facial hairs such as those on the upper lip and chin. Will last 4 to 5 weeks.

- **Waxing/Threading/Sugaring:** Best for eyebrows and any dark facial hair. Removes all hair in the area treated. Will last 5 to 6 weeks.

- **Electrolysis:** Works by transmitting an electric current along the shaft of each hair and killing the hair follicle to stop regrowth. It is expensive and can be uncomfortable, but if done properly, it will give permanent results. Some stubborn hairs may need to have the treatment repeated.

- **Laser treatment:** In many instances, laser hair removal has replaced electrolysis, as it is less painful. It works by passing a beam of light down the hair shaft and destroying the hair follicle, again to stop regrowth. Because of the use of light, it is more effective on dark hairs and may not be effective on blond hairs. Seek professional advice.

LEFT **A trip to your beauty salon not only improves the appearance of your skin but is relaxing and gives you a feeling of well-being, too.**

FACIAL WORKOUT

A few facial stretches and a gentle workout can do wonders for toning your facial muscles. The exercises below form a facial workout that will only take 5 minutes and should be repeated every day. Try to find a regular time slot such as after your morning skincare routine, while watching television, or whenever you have a spare moment to devote to yourself.

Chin toner

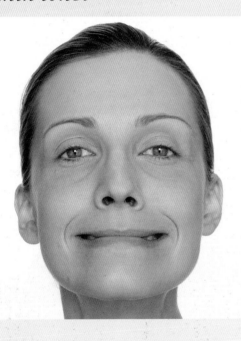

The Chin Toner helps prevent jowls. Gently bring your teeth up to rest on your top lip with your head tilted slightly backward and your chin thrust forward. Start to smile slowly, hold for a count of 5, and then relax slowly, bringing your mouth back to its normal position. Repeat twice and you will feel the muscles around your neck and jaw pull slightly.

Eye drainage

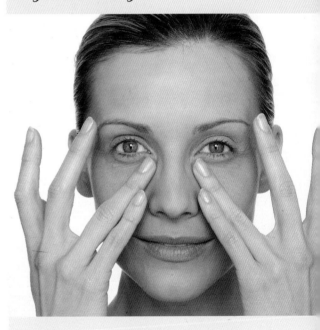

This exercise stimulates lymphatic drainage around the eye area and helps reduce puffiness. Looking straight ahead, and using your ring finger, gently tap along the eyebrow, starting at the inner end and working outward. Continue to tap your finger along the top of the cheekbones and then up the sides of the nostrils ending back at the eyebrow.

Smile lift

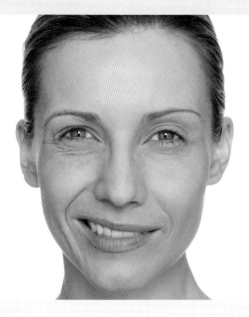

The Smile Lift helps to tone the muscles around the mouth and firm the cheeks. With a relaxed bite, look into a mirror and smile on one side of your mouth, pulling your mouth up as far as it will go. Hold for a count of 5, relax slowly, and repeat on the other side.

Eye lift

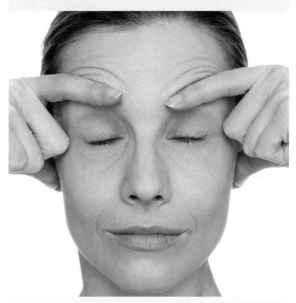

This exercise helps reduce frown lines. Curve your index fingers along your eyebrows and gently push upward. Hold your fingers firmly against your forehead, looking straight ahead. Close your eyes very slowly, feeling them pull downward away from the brow. Squeeze very tightly and hold for a count of 5. Relax slowly and repeat twice more.

Frown pinch

The Frown Pinch will help soften visible lines. Relax your face, then, using your index finger and thumb, gently pinch any frown lines you have on your forehead —these may by vertical or horizontal. The pinching will increase blood flow.

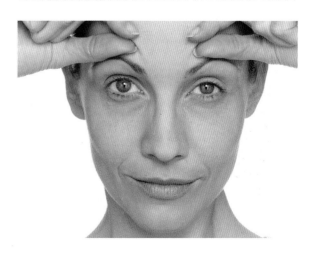

SUN CARE

Although a tan may make us feel like we look healthy and younger, UV rays account for most of our skin's premature aging, including wrinkles and age spots. Sun exposure is also hazardous and can have more serious effects than premature aging, most notably causing skin cancer. However, with a little sun sense you can enjoy the rays without risking your skin.

Sunlight is an important source of vitamin D, which our body needs for, among other things, healthy bones and teeth. Just 10 minutes of sunshine can prevent vitamin D deficiency: morning is a good time when the UV rays are weaker. Avoid overexposure to the sun and use caution by wearing a sunscreen with a Sun Protection Factor (SPF) of 15 or higher on a daily basis, throughout the year. Choose a facial moisturizer with SPF for everyday protection. However, if you are out in the sun for long periods, or sunbathing, use an additional sunscreen with SPF 30 or higher.

SIMPLE SUN SAFETY

Being aware of the strength of the sun and taking simple preventive measures, such as covering up with clothing and sunglasses, will reduce the risk of exposure. Avoid being in the sun between 10 a.m. and 2 p.m., when the UV rays are strongest. If you're spending time in the sun, keep these guidelines in mind:

APPLYING SUNSCREEN

No sunscreen, whether it's factor 15 or 50, will give the protection you need unless it's applied properly. Apply to clean, dry skin at least half an hour before exposure —it takes about this long to be properly absorbed. Always apply cream or lotion liberally to completely cover all areas that will be exposed and don't over-massage it in. Reapply regularly—sunscreen can easily be sweated, washed or rubbed off—every 2 hours in the sun or immediately after excessive sweating or swimming (even "waterproof" sunscreens need to be reapplied after you've been in the water).

Apply sunscreen anywhere your skin is exposed— hands and décolletage are particularly vulnerable.

SUNSCREEN KNOW-HOW

A higher SPF doesn't mean that you can stay out in the sun longer, just that it filters out more UV rays. For your sunscreen to be effective it needs to be stored properly: do not store sunscreens in hot places or allow

BELOW When out in the sun, choose SPF 30 or higher; the higher the numbers, the better the protection against UVA and UVB rays.

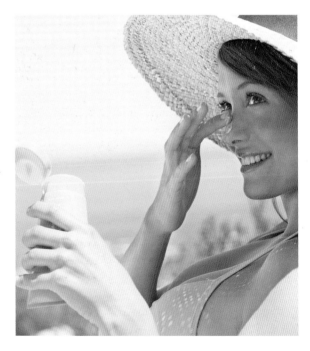

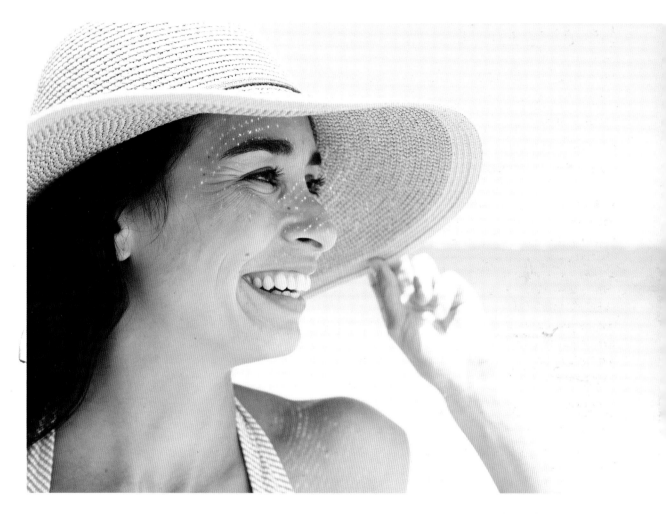

them to overheat in the sun, as the heat can ruin their protective ingredients. Check the expiration date on your sunscreen before you use it—most sunscreens have a shelf life of 1 to 2 years and after this time won't be as effective.

SENSITIVE SKIN

For sensitive skin, look for sunblocks containing titanium dioxide, which blocks out the UV rays. Avoid sunscreen with chemical sun filters that start a reaction in the skin once they are exposed to the sun, as they may irritate. Tan accelerators are ideal for those who suffer with heat rash (hives) or burn easily. They prepare the

ABOVE Covering your head with a broad-brimmed hat is a great way to block the harsh rays of the sun from your eyes and face.

skin for exposure to the sun by stimulating its natural melanin, thereby prolonging the tan while also softening and moisturizing the skin.

SKINCARE TIP

After exposure, use an after-sun product with cooling properties, such as aloe vera, or a rich moisturizer to replenish and hydrate the skin.

APPLYING
MAKE-UP

The cosmetic counters abound with products. Magazines are full of tips and ideas. Where do you start? What do you do with all those different tubes and jars? The following pages will guide you through this plethora of choice, from the essential tools and equipment that will ensure a professional look, to straightforward advice on each product and how best to apply it to get a flawless finish every time. Inspired and informed, your next trip to the beauty counter will be as pleasurable as it should be.

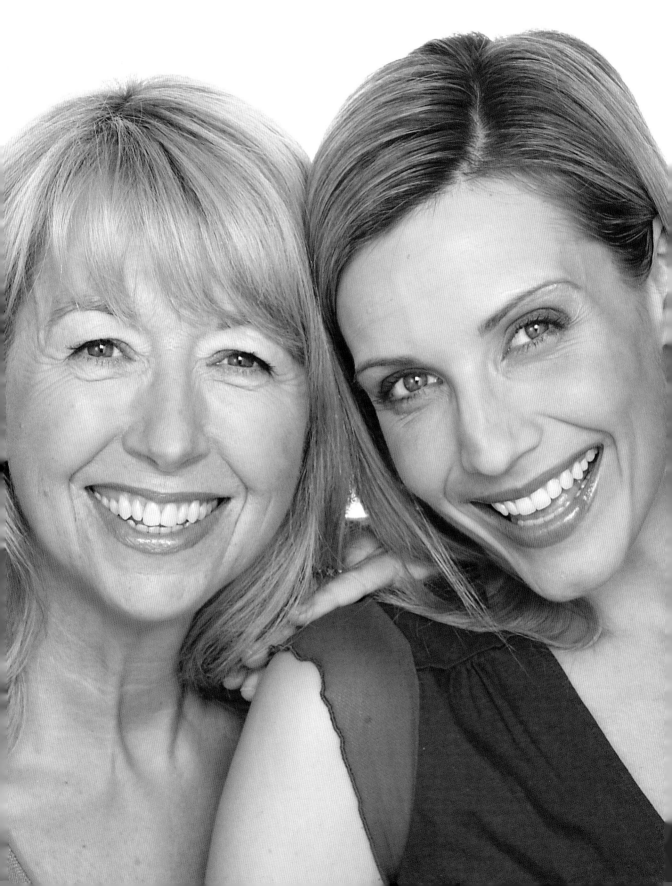

TOOLS OF THE TRADE

A perfect make-up cannot be achieved without the right tools—brushes, sponges, eyelash curlers—all form a key part of your routine and will help you achieve your make-up's full potential. Investing in a quality set of basic make-up tools will pay dividends—application will be easier and the tools themselves will last longer.

BRUSHES

When selecting your brushes, make sure the ferrule that holds the bristles together is crimped and tight to hold the bristles in, and that the bristles texture is soft.

- **Powder brush**: A big, fluffy brush used to whisk off excess loose powder or for applying bronzer.

- **Blush brush**: A medium-full, round brush used to apply a concentration of color.

- **Foundation brush**: Similar to a painter's brush, this has soft bristles held tightly together, which makes applying liquid foundation a breeze.

- **Eyebrow brush**: Stiff bristles to blend and a comb to shape the eyebrows.

- **Blender brush**: A soft, fluffy brush to take the edge off color that is used for applying highlighter and blending eye shadows.

- **Angled brush**: Tapered edges allow the middle bristles to position the eye shadow accurately when applying contouring and accent eye shadows. By dampening the bristles, you can also use this brush to apply eye shadow as eye liner.

- **Concealer brush**: A narrow, firm brush with a flat head that is best used in a dabbing motion.

- **Lip brush**: Should be small and firm. Provides a more effective and longer application of lipstick than simply applying lipstick on its own. Look for a retractable version for cleanliness and portability.

ESSENTIAL TOOLS

In addition to your brushes, you will need a few items to help apply, correct, remove, and improve your make-up. To keep your tools clean and hygienic either wash or dispose of them regularly (see pages 32–33).

- **Tweezers**: Metal ones with flat ends tend to have a better grip for extracting unwanted hairs.

- **Eyelash curlers**: Choose metal rather than plastic. This scissorlike apparatus has rubber pads that press on the lashes, giving them extra lift and curl. They are usually only used on upper lashes and can be used before or after mascara application.

- **Sponges**: Come in many shapes, although wedge tends to be the best for blending in foundation and getting into the crevices around the nose and eyes.

- **Velour powder puff**: Used to press on face powder to give a smooth finish and keep foundation in place.

- **Cotton pads**: Disposable pads used for removing eye make-up and cleansers and for applying toner and loose powder.

- **Cotton swabs**: Dip the tip of the swab in foundation or make-up remover to tidy up any make-up smudges or mistakes.

- **Pencil sharpeners**: Make sure to purchase one designed especially for eye and lip pencils, which can accommodate the soft lead. An ordinary pencil sharpener will break the soft lead.

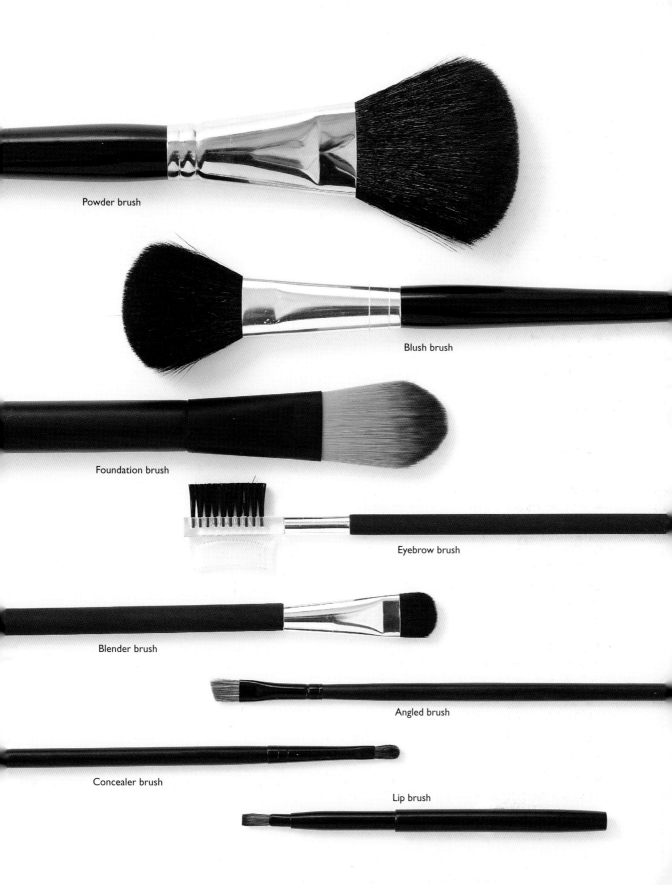

Powder brush

Blush brush

Foundation brush

Eyebrow brush

Blender brush

Angled brush

Concealer brush

Lip brush

CARING FOR YOUR PRODUCTS

We all have it—a heavy make-up bag with products that have been there for years and years. We kid ourselves that they will come in handy one day, but in reality they end up being a nuisance, and a cumbersome and unhygienic one at that. Organizing, cleaning, and sorting your tools and products will kick-start a new look and freshen up your make-up in more ways than one.

Start by gathering all of your products, from your dressing table or bathroom cabinet to your make-up bag, and place them on a flat surface. Throw out anything that is two years old or more. Smell everything —if it has an unusual or musty odor, toss it.

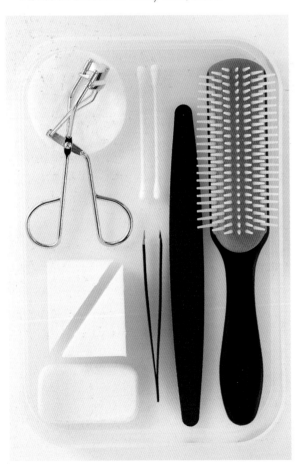

SHELF LIFE

Check the shelf life of any remaining products. The longer you keep a product, the more it is exposed to the air; and the more you touch it, the less hygienic, clean, and effective it becomes.

Most packaging will either have use-by dates or "period after opening" timelines, indicated by an open jar with the number of months beside it. Throw them out if you know they've outlived their shelf life.

Keep the following life spans in mind (from the time they are first opened):

- **Mascara and liquid eye liners:** 3 months
- **Lipstick and lip gloss:** 1 year
- **Foundation and concealer:** 1 year
- **Pencils (eye, eyebrow, lip):** 18 months (sharpen to remove the top layer, which can get dirty)
- **Cream eye shadows and blush:** 18 months
- **Powders, eye shadows, blush, bronzers:** 2 years

TOOLS

Good hygiene is crucial, not only to ensure that your investment tools work their best, but also to prevent breakouts and infections.

LEFT Keeping your tools in a separate container to your make-up will prevent them picking up loose powders or dust.

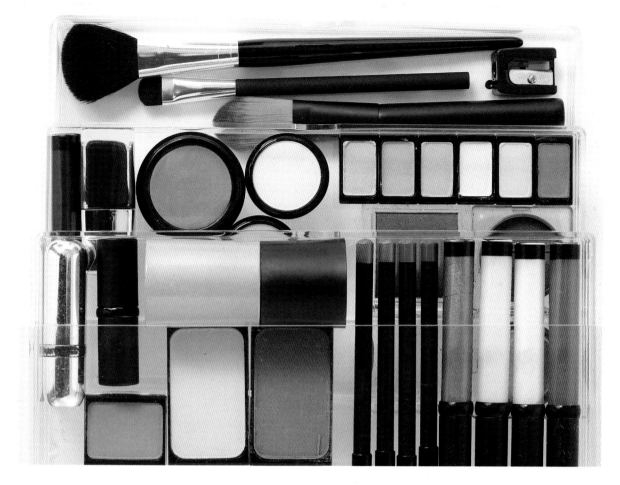

ABOVE Plexiglas organizers are a great way to store make-up and tools, as everything is clearly visible.

- **Make-up brushes** should be washed regularly, at least once a month, using a brush cleanser or mild shampoo. Cup your hand, fill it with warm, soapy water, and swirl the brush in your palm until clean. Rinse well, then squeeze any excess water from the brush. Leave the brush to air-dry overnight by lying it down over the edge of a table so that the bristles are open to the air.

- **Disposable sponges** should be replaced once soiled, or washed daily.

- **Velour sponges** should be washed weekly and replaced every 6 months.

- **Eyelash curler rubber pads** should be replaced regularly, every 2 months. Clean eyelash curlers, tweezers, and pencil sharpeners with a few drops of tea-tree oil every couple of months.

STORING YOUR PRODUCTS

Make sure that your products are sealed tight and stored out of sunlight, which can destroy the preservatives. Some women like to store their make-up in drawers with dividers, while others prefer to use Plexiglas organizers so that they can see everything.

Find a system that works for you, but make sure that it isn't "all thrown into a bag"—you'll never be able to find anything, and most of it will go unused.

It's also a good idea to have two make-up kits. One for home and a smaller one for your handbag or when you are on the go.

BEAUTY TIP

Never share your tools, brushes, or cosmetics with others.

CREATING A FLAWLESS FINISH

The first step in your make-up routine is to create a flawless finish for your face. Depending on the season, your age, the occasion, and even your health, you will need to use a variety of products, either on their own or in conjunction with each other, to create a natural look. Assess what each product does and see if will work for you.

Foundation, in its many forms, prepares a smooth and even base. Once you have applied the right foundation, you will be ready to apply make-up to your eyes, cheeks, and finally, lips.

SKIN PRIMERS

These come in a variety of formats, designed to smooth out the surface of the skin and even out skin tone. Skin primers are always lighter in consistency than concealers, so are best used after your moisturizer and under foundation. They are perfect for hiding dark circles and blemishes, especially near the eyes.

PRIMERS THAT SMOOTH

These are usually neutral in color and give the skin an even and silky finish. Use this type of primer to boost dull skin if there is a lack of sunshine, it's the wrong time of the month. or any time you feel your skin lacks luster.

PRIMERS THAT EVEN OUT SKIN TONE

Normally available in three shades: yellow, lavender, and mint green. Each is designed to correct a particular skin tone, giving it an even appearance:

- **Yellow** will generally reduce mild pinkness and dark circles under the eyes. It can also be applied to fine lines to reduce their appearance.

- **Lavender** is a wonderful lift for sallow skin or if you are feeling under the weather and looking vaguely jaundiced. It counteracts yellow tones and helps illuminate the skin.

- **Mint** is a pale green primer that counteracts any redness in the skin tone. It will immediately help conceal any rosy tones, and is especially good if you suffer from rosacea (see page 21). You will need to apply foundation and powder over it to stop the green tones from showing through.

FOUNDATION

Finding a foundation that suits your skin and lifestyle is all-important. There are many formulas, but they all have one thing in common—they should give your skin an even colour.

- **Tinted moisturizers** are the lightest foundations. They are great for young skin and in the summer when you have a tan and want lighter coverage. Tinted moisturizers don't cover blemishes or pimples, but they will even out skin tone.

- **Liquid or fluid foundations** will give more coverage. They are slightly more difficult to apply and must match your skin tone, otherwise they will be noticeable around the jawline.

- **Cream or stick foundation** is the heaviest formulation and is good for those with less-than-perfect skin who love a made-up look.

CHOOSING YOUR FOUNDATION

If you wear foundation every day, make sure it has a good SPF, which will give you added protection against sun damage (see pages 26–27).

Test the color on your jawline, not your hand, cheek, or wrist. The right color will vanish into the skin. Always test in daylight and, if in a store, ask for a hand mirror and take it outside. You may need one color for summer and a lighter one for winter. You can blend the two in the transitional seasons.

MINERAL POWDERS

These lightweight loose powder foundations are an alternative to cream or liquid foundations. They give the skin a smooth, natural finish and are especially good for younger skin types who may be sensitive to oil-based liquid foundations. They brush onto the skin, and can be built up in layers for medium coverage. Many also provide everyday SPF sun protection.

LOOSE POWDER

Professional make-up artists always finish their make-up with an application of loose powder, often applying many layers. Loose powder will ensure a long-lasting, matte look, which may not be to everyone's taste. You may prefer to carry a pressed powder in your handbag to simply control any shine while you are on the go.

CONCEALERS

Concealers are always best used over foundation, as their consistency may be up to five times heavier. Use them as a last resort to cover blemishes and dark circles. If you need to apply concealer near the eye, blend with your eye cream for a softer application and so that it won't settle into any lines.

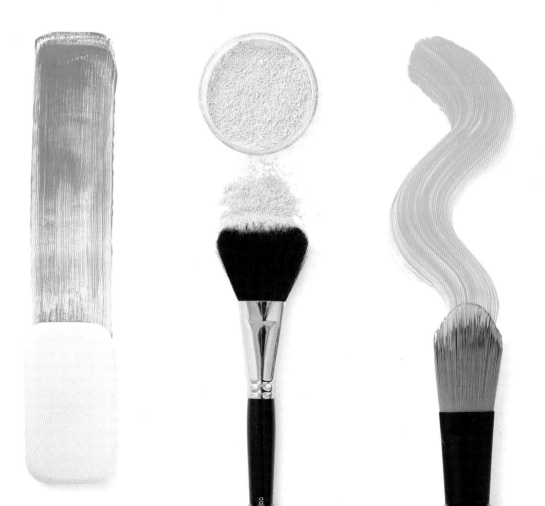

Applying primer **YOU WILL NEED** *primer, foundation brush, concealer brush or sponge*

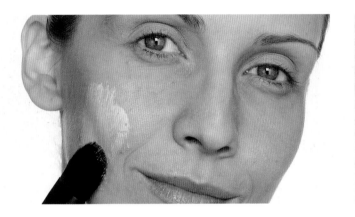

Smoothing primer

Apply all over the face using a foundation brush, fingertips or sponge. The effect will even out the skin's surface and make pores appear smaller.

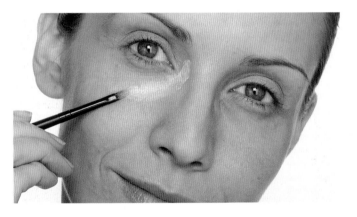

Coloured primers for dark shadows under the eyes

After applying an eye gel, use a small sponge, or concealer or foundation brush to apply the primer gently around the eye area to hide dark circles or shadows. Make sure to also apply right in the corner of the eye, near the nose, which can often be very blue in colour.

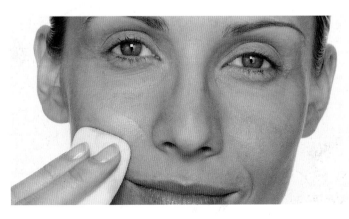

Coloured primers for evening out skin tone

After the application of your moisturizer, apply the primer to all the areas on the face that are uneven in tone. Using a sponge or foundation brush, gently dab the primer on, rather than rubbing into the skin, which will lessen its effectiveness.

Applying foundation **YOU WILL NEED** *foundation, foundation brush*

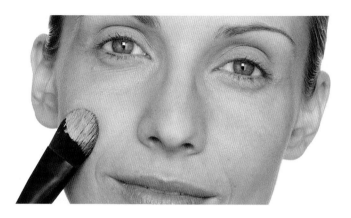

Start applying the foundation to either cheek, dabbing it on using gentle tapping movements with a sponge, or short strokes with a foundation brush. Do not dot the foundation onto the face, as this will cause it to dry unevenly.

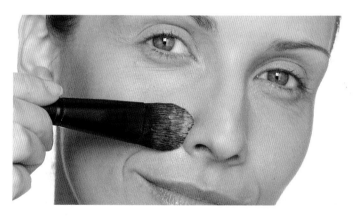

Move to the nose, making sure you get into the creases around the nostrils, then apply to the chin and finally the forehead. Blend gently out toward the edge of the face and hairline. Do not apply to eyelids.

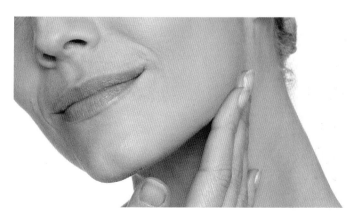

Finally, check in the mirror to make sure there is no defined line around the jaw and that your foundation is evenly applied all over.

Applying concealer YOU WILL NEED *concealer, concealer brush*

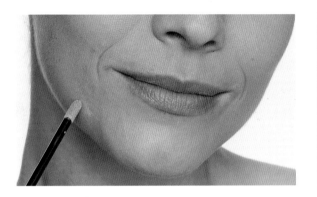

Be sure to choose a color of concealer that blends with your foundation. Use either the applicator it comes with or a concealer brush. Dab the concealer lightly on the area you want to hide and blend the edges. For concealing blemishes or dark spots, cream or stick concealers give the best coverage.

Applying mineral powder YOU WILL NEED *mineral powder, powder brush*

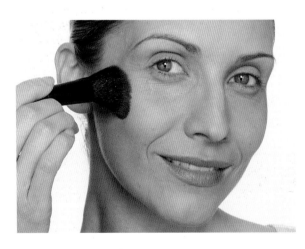

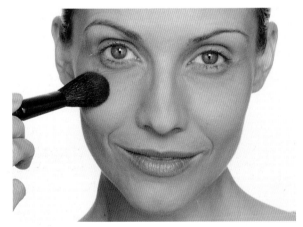

1 Use a firm, round-ended brush. Place a small amount of powder in the lid of the container, to avoid uneven coverage. After coating the brush in powder, tap it against a hard surface to knock off any excess, and apply to small areas of the face at a time in a circular motion.

2 Apply a second layer, building up the coverage as you go. You may need to use a finer brush to apply to smaller areas. Mineral powder can also be used as a concealer or to hide dark circles under the eyes.

Applying loose powder YOU WILL NEED *loose powder, powder brush*

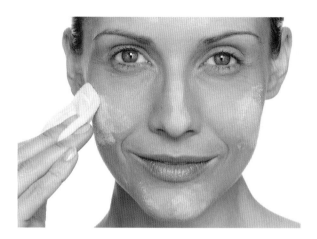

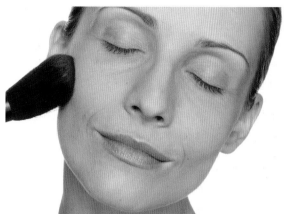

Tip loose powder into its lid, enough to apply to the skin. Use the powder puff supplied with the product to generously apply the powder all over the face, avoiding the soft skin tissue around the eye area, which might attract too much powder and exacerbate fine lines and wrinkles.

With a large powder brush, start at the top of the face and use downward strokes to brush off any excess powder. This will leave a smooth surface, ensuring that any facial hair will lie flat.

Applying pressed powder YOU WILL NEED *pressed powder, cotton pad*

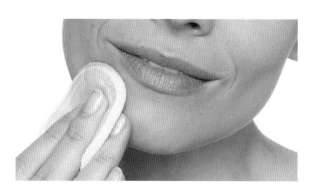

Pressed powder may be applied with the powder puff supplied with the product or a cotton pad. Make sure the powder puff is absolutely clean, as these pads tend to become clogged with foundation from previous applications. Press the powder firmly onto the skin. If there is any excess, turn the pad over and whisk it off.

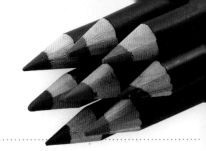

MAKING UP YOUR EYES

With a flawless complexion, you are now ready to add some definition to your look, starting with your eyes. The art of good eye make-up is to enhance the eyes' color and shape. By using the correct products in the right way, you will find your eye make-up routine a pleasure rather than a chore.

EYE BASE

An eye base will make your eye shadow stay in place all day without creasing or smudging. It will also protect the skin on your eye from discoloring due to the pigmentation in the shadows. Apply using your ring finger.

EYE SHADOWS

Available in a huge palette of colors and finishes, eye shadows come in two main formulations:

- **Cream eye shadows** are quick to apply and give a more subtle look. Creams can slide and gather in the creases, and are not ideal for oily skin.

- **Powder eye shadows** tend to come in a greater variety of shades and have finishes from matte to shimmer and frosted. Choose finely milled powders that feel smooth to the touch rather than dusty ones, which can look cakey and exaggerate lines.

EYE PENCILS

Used to define the eye along the lashes with a soft line. Rather than the traditional black, which is often too harsh and can, in fact, make the eye look smaller, choose from a variety of colors that suit your personal coloring.

LIQUID EYE LINER

This is a liquid that is applied to the eye with a fine brush. It gives a strong look and is great for dramatic eyes or for extending the line around the eye. It takes a lot of practice to get it right, but the finished effect can be stunning.

MASCARA

If you apply nothing else before you leave the house, apply your mascara—it immediately gives definition to the eyes.

There are hundreds of different types available, from lash-building ones that attach fibers to the lashes to conditioning ones that feed and nourish. Choose a color that will work with your natural coloring:

- **Black brown** is flattering on most types.

- **Black** is good for Deeps and Clears.

- **Mid or warm brown** looks great on Lights, Warms and Softs.

- **Navy** mascaras look good on Cools—but be careful not to distract from your natural eye color.

- **Colored** mascaras are fun for special occasions.

EYEBROW PENCILS

Your eyebrows are the frame for your eyes, but are often forgotten. Using a pencil to define or color sparse eyebrows will complete your look. Eyebrow pencils are firmer than an eye pencil, which needs to be soft for ease of application. Choose a color close to your hair color, and your brows will look natural.

BEAUTY TIP

Never pump your mascara wand—this will force air into the tube, which will dry it out.

Applying eye shadow **YOU WILL NEED** *eye base, blender brush, angled brush, eye shadows (base, contour, accent, blender shades)*

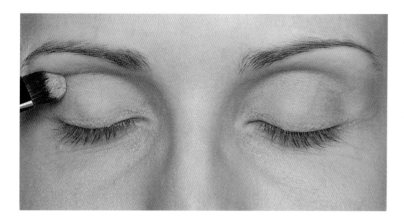

After applying an eye base, choose one of the lightest neutral colors from your eye shadow palette, and with the blender brush apply over the entire eye area. The base color, also known as the highlight shade, will ensure that additional colors will blend together.

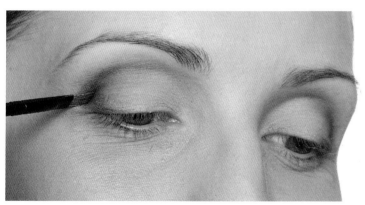

Next, take the angled brush and apply a neutral, medium-depth color, known as a contour shade, if you want to shade or contour any area of the eye. Now apply the strongest or accent color using the same brush to give the eye definition.

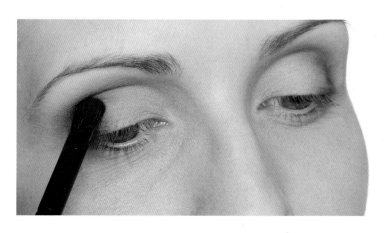

Using the blender brush and your blender shade, which should also be a medium, neutral-depth shade, blend all the colors together to give an even look all over. This will prevent any blocks of color or harsh edges between the contour shade and accent colour.

Applying eye pencil YOU WILL NEED *eye pencil*

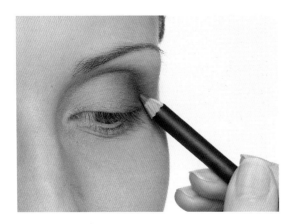

1 Start with the pencil at the outer edge of the top lash line. Look down and draw a fine line inward as close to the lash as possible. If the eyelid is a little crêpey, lift the eyebrow to stretch the skin. Always lift up, never out, which can damage the fine tissue around the eye. If you find this difficult, gently hold down the eyelid with two fingertips either side and draw a line (with the other hand) from the outside in. Try not to draw the other way, as you can end up with an uneven line.

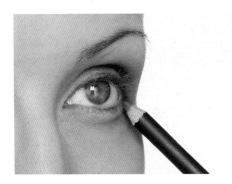

2 Now look up and draw a fine line underneath the lower lash line, halfway along, again starting from the outside of the eye and working inward. Outlining the eye completely with eye pencil can make the eye look even smaller. If the line is too harsh, use a cotton swab to soften, or apply eye shadow over the top.

Applying liquid eye liner YOU WILL NEED *liquid eye liner*

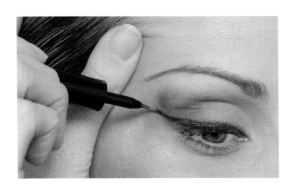

Lift the eye at the eyebrow and, looking down, start painting the liner on with the brush. Start from the outer edge of the eye, as the liquid is more likely to smudge or appear uneven if you start from the inside of the eye. Line the top lid first, then the lower lid. If you want to extend the line, start at the outer corner of the eye and wing gently upward.

Applying mascara YOU WILL NEED *mascara*

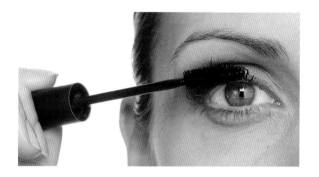

Look straight ahead and brush the mascara along the lashes, turning the brush as you go. To create extra thickness, hold the wand horizontally at the base of the lashes and wiggle it back and forth before drawing it up and out to the tip. If you want to apply mascara to the lower lashes, hold the mascara wand vertically and use just the tip of the brush.

Applying eyebrow pencil YOU WILL NEED *eyebrow brush, eyebrow pencil*

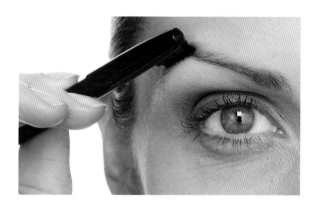

Use an eyebrow brush to remove any trace of make-up (foundation, powder, or eye shadow), brushing the brows the wrong way, then brush the brows into shape, making sure all the hairs are lying flat.

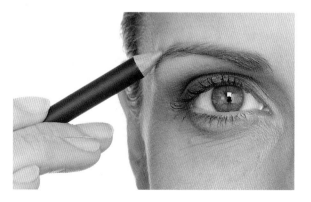

Use a blonde pencil for fair brows and a brown one for darker brows and draw tiny, feathery strokes on the skin to give definition to the eye. See page 110 for tips on how to enhance your eyebrows further.

MAKING UP YOUR CHEEKS

A hint of color on your cheeks gives a healthy, natural look to your make-up. Blush can be used to enhance your face shape (see pages 102–107) and becomes more important the older we get, as the cheeks tend to flatten. An eye-catching touch of blush can illuminate the cheekbones and draw the eye upward.

There are many different forms of blush and bronzers, but to make your blush last longer, choose one that is the same texture as your foundation.

POWDER BLUSH

This long-lasting blush works well on all skin types, and is excellent if you have oily skin, but not so good in hot weather on a perspiring skin as it may run. Always apply with a blush brush. Sweep the brush across the powder and, before applying to the face, give it a tap on your hand to remove any excess. Natural tones are best, but if you have dark skin you'll need a bright blush.

CREAM BLUSH

Quick and easy to apply, cream blush is great for those with dry skin. Apply on the apples of your cheeks to mimic the flush you get from exercising, but be aware that this will bring attention to your nose. You can put cream blush straight onto the skin if you have good natural color and are not wearing foundation.

BRONZER

Bronzers are becoming increasingly popular either for contouring the face or as a blush on darker skin tones. Alternatively, you can simply brush a bronzer on eyelids and cheeks for a speedy glow if you don't have time for a full make-up. For a great look on a tanned skin, put your bronzer where the sun naturally hits your face—on the center of your forehead, cheekbones, and chin. Women with darker skin tones often find bronzers work better than colored blush.

IRIDESCENT HIGHLIGHTERS

Iridescent highlighters draw attention to the eye and should be used in conjunction with blushes or bronzers to balance the effect. They can be powder, cream, or liquid based. Careful, well-blended application is needed to give a subtle effect, when using cream or powder, so only apply on areas that you want highlighted, such as the inner corners of your eye, under your brow bones, or your cupid's bow (the center of your lips).

Applying cream blush
YOU WILL NEED *cream blush*

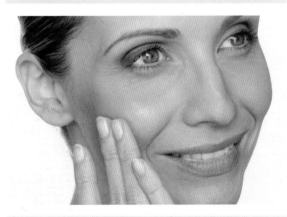

Warm the blush, either between your fingertips or on the back of your hand, then press onto the cheeks so it melts into the skin. If using on skin without a foundation base, apply a primer or moisturizer first.

Applying powder blush YOU WILL NEED *powder blush, blush brush*

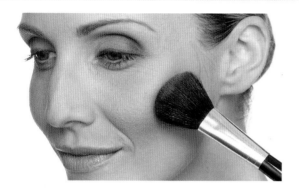

Load your blush brush with powder blush (see page 44). To enhance your face shape, apply along the cheekbones and out toward the temples, then work the brush around in circles to give a soft edge. For a fun and youthful look, apply to the apple of the cheeks. This is not advised, however, if you blush easily, have any broken capillaries, have close-set eyes, or are trying to draw attention away from a large nose.

Applying bronzer YOU WILL NEED *bronzer, powder brush*

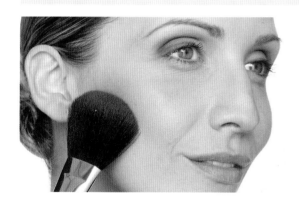

Load your powder brush with either pressed or loose powder bronzer, then whisk the brush over the areas where your face would normally catch the sun—along the cheekbones, forehead, bridge of the nose and chin. Use with caution and do not overapply, as it can give the appearance of dirty skin.

Applying iridescent highlighter YOU WILL NEED *iridescent highlighter*

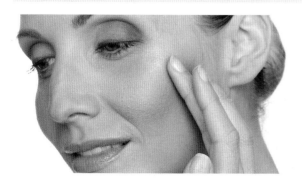

To enhance your bone structure, use the iridescent highlighter's applicator or your fingertips to apply in a "C" shape, starting at the temples and then outward and along the cheekbones for the most impact. For darker skin tones, mix iridescent highlighters and bronzers together.

MAKING UP YOUR LIPS

No other products are more widely used by women than lipstick and lip gloss. They are quickly applied, with or without a mirror, depending on your skills, and have an instant effect, giving color to your face and turning your look from day to night with a simple change of shade. Making them last, though, is a matter of proper application and the use of different products.

LIP BASE

Applying a lip base or lip primer will ensure that your lipstick has some staying power and the color will be purer. It also helps stop lip colors from bleeding into the fine lines around the mouth. The majority of lip bases contain ingredients such as avocado oil, which help moisturize the lips.

LIP PENCILS

A selection of colored pencils can greatly extend the shades you can use on your lips. Your lip pencil can tone with your choice of lipstick or you can achieve a completely different look with different shades: a red pencil with a pink lipstick will have a stronger appearance while using a natural shade with a brighter lipstick will tone the lipstick shade down. Lip pencils can also be used to help correct an uneven-shaped mouth and balance the lips (see page 111), if necessary.

LIPSTICKS

Lipsticks come in many formulations, with varying degrees of pigmentation and lasting qualities. Matte lipsticks have the greatest pigmentation and often feel dry on the lips but last longer. Sheer lipsticks are halfway between a gloss and a cream, and will feel softer on the mouth. Shimmery lipsticks have light-reflecting properties that help make lips look fuller.

LIP GLOSS

The sales of lip gloss have overtaken those of lipstick in the last decade, mainly due to their ease of application and moisturizing qualities. Lip glosses can be used on their own, on top of a lip pencil, or over a matte or cream lipstick to give a shimmery or glossy finish. For a long-lasting look, layering your lip products is the answer. Lip stains have recently been added to make-up counters. They have true staying power, but the disadvantage is that, once applied, it is difficult to change the color.

BEAUTY TIP

To stop your lipstick from ending up on your teeth, place a clean index finger between your lips and pull it out. Any lipstick that was on the inside of your lips will end up on your finger.

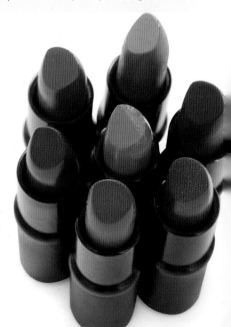

Applying lip base YOU WILL NEED *lip base, lip brush*

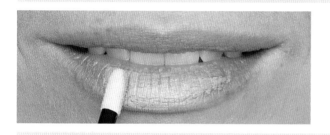

Smile while applying a small amount of the base with its own applicator, or a lip brush, to distribute evenly and smoothly. Allow to dry for 15 seconds before applying lipstick.

Applying lip pencil YOU WILL NEED *lip pencil*

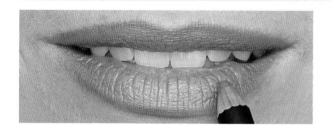

Using the tip of the pencil, outline the whole mouth to stop the lipstick from bleeding. Then, using the side of the point of the pencil, fill in the rest of the lips to give color and depth to your lipstick or gloss.

Applying lipstick YOU WILL NEED *lipstick, lip brush, tissue*

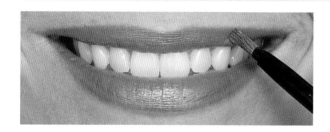

Load your lip brush and work the lipstick thoroughly into the bristles of the brush. Smile and apply lipstick all over the lips. Blot with a tissue, reapply and blot again to remove any excess grease from the lipstick.

Applying lip gloss YOU WILL NEED *lip gloss, lip brush*

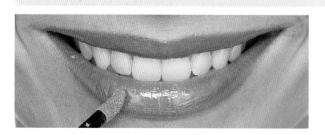

Using either its own applicator or a lip brush, apply your lip gloss on top of lipstick. Alternatively, to give the illusion of plumper lips, try applying just to the center of the mouth.

IDENTIFYING
YOUR COLORING

Understanding your coloring is the next step in helping you achieve a perfect make-up look. The aim is to create balance and harmony between your natural coloring and the colors of clothes and make-up you wear. By wearing the right make-up colors, you will not only feel good but look younger, healthier, and fitter. Your hair, eye, and skin tone may change over time, so remember to be honest and positive about yourself and have fun discovering your coloring type.

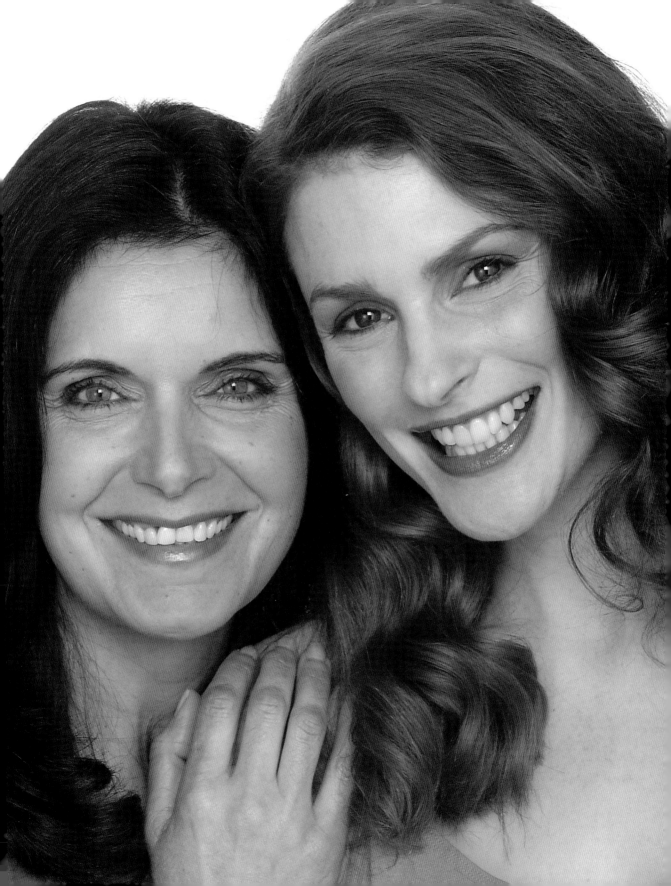

THE RIGHT COLORS FOR YOU

Your make-up should complement your natural coloring and the clothes that you wear to create a balanced and harmonious look. To help you make the right decisions, we have devised a system of six general coloring types, and will guide you through the best make-up colours for you. A little background color theory will help you put this advice into practise.

UNDERSTANDING COLOR

We have based our principles of color analysis on the Munsell Color System. It is one of the most useful and universally recognized because it organizes colors logically. Munsell used three terms to describe color: hue, value, and chroma.

HUE (UNDERTONE: WARM OR COOL)

Hue defines whether a color is warm (yellow-based) or cool (blue-based). All colors can be described as having either a warm or cool undertone. For example, a coral lipstick has a yellow undertone, therefore will be a warm shade, whereas a plum lipstick has a blue undertone, so it will be considered a cool shade.

VALUE (DEPTH: LIGHT OR DEEP)

The value of color refers to its depth, giving a measure of how light or dark a color is. All colors can have a range of depth—for example, blue eye shadows can go from very pale blue to dark navy. Depending on your coloring type, you can decide what depth of coloring suits you best.

CHROMA (CLARITY: SOFT OR CLEAR)

Chroma indicates the purity or clarity of a color. Some colors are bright and vibrant, while others are more muted or dusty. Clear, bright colors, such as a teal-colored eye pencil, will attract attention to the eye, whereas a softer coffee-colored pencil, for example, will have a more subtle and muted quality to it.

PERSONAL COLORING

The aim of color analysis is to create harmony between your own coloring and the make-up colors you wear. This is achieved by wearing colors whose characteristics are the same as or similar to your own coloring, based on a combination of hair color, eye color and skin tone.

Analyze your personal characteristics to discover your dominant coloring type: Light, Deep, Warm, Cool, Clear, or Soft (see pages 52–75 to identify which one you are) and the appropriate colors that will give a harmonious and balanced look to your make-up.

YOUR BEST MAKE-UP COLORS

There are thousands of shades of make-up colors out there—some will make you look radiant, while others can make you look unhealthy or age you prematurely. Once you understand your coloring type and your best make-up colors, you can limit the cosmetics that you buy, buying only those that will make you look fabulous, and come up with some wonderful color combinations. Best of all, the recommended make-up colors will work with your wardrobe, too.

COLOR TIP

If you've had a color analysis in the past, be aware that over time your characteristics may change—look at yourself as you are today.

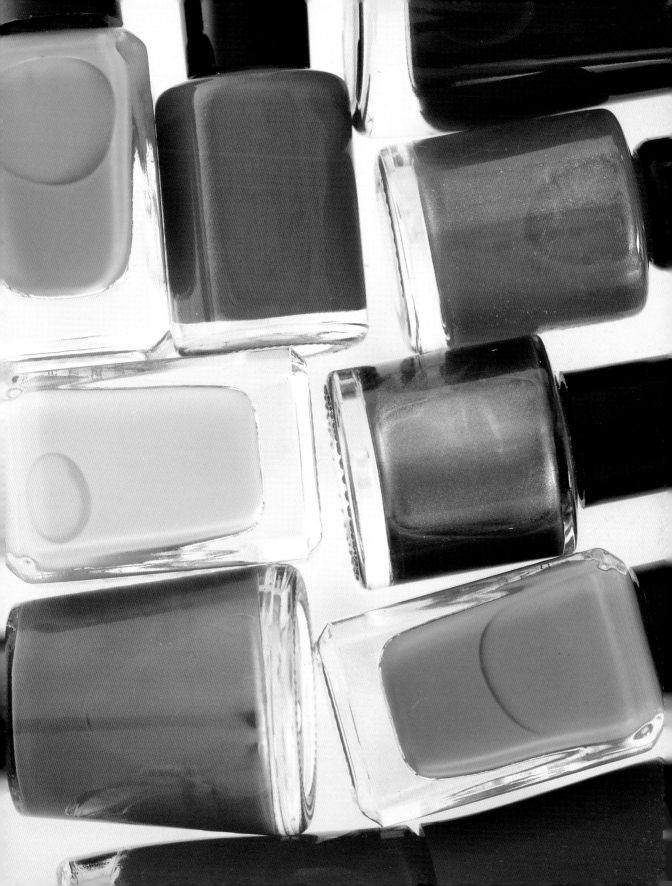

LIGHT

Your overall look is pale and delicate. The undertone of your coloring can be warm, with golden tints to your hair and a few freckles on your skin, or cool, with ash tones to your hair and a slight pinkish tint to your skin. Because of your delicate coloring you need to be cautious with your make-up palette so that the colors do not overpower the light tones of your hair and eyes.

ARE YOU A LIGHT?

Do you have…?

- Indistinguishable, pale eyebrows (that you may tint or pencil in to give definition)
- Pale eyelashes (that you may tint)
- Pale blue, pale green, or pale brown eyes
- Naturally blonde or very light hair
- A pale or porcelain complexion

MAKE-UP GUIDELINES

- **Face:** Take particular care when choosing your foundation or tinted moisturizer so that it tones in perfectly with your complexion. Test it against your jawline to see if it blends in well. Don't be tempted by a foundation that is a few shades darker than your natural skin tone, as this can be aging, and it is difficult to make it look natural.

- **Eyes:** By all means tint your lashes and brows to a medium brown color (rather than dark brown or black), which will alleviate the necessity to overapply mascara and eyebrow pencil. Keep your eye shadow shades light to medium in depth, so as not to distract from the gorgeous pale color of your eyes. If you have pale green or very pale brown eyes, soft brown eye pencils will be best; for pale blue eyes, a teal eye pencil will really make your eyes pop.

- **Cheeks:** Lighter shades of blush will be much more flattering than deep tones. Try not to overapply it either; a simple whisk with your blush brush over the cheeks is all your delicate coloring needs.

- **Lips:** Avoid dark colors, even if they are fashionable. If you have freckles, try coral or peachy lip pencils, lipsticks, or glosses. If you have more of a pinkish tone to your skin, go for a light rose lip shade instead.

WEARING COLOR

Because of your light and delicate coloring, you need to always wear a light color near your face. Avoid dark colors, which will overpower your lovely porcelain look. If you need to wear darker colors—for example. if you work in a formal environment—make sure you pair them with a light-colored top or scarf. Tonal colors will also look good on you, especially for a more formal or professional look. Avoid black-and-white combinations, which will overpower your delicate coloring. In warmer weather, you will look great wearing two light colors together. Or, if wearing just one color, make sure it's either light or medium in depth. Black will make you look older than your years, and for you is not slimming. There are many great alternatives, such as greys, light navies, medium browns, and taupes.

ACCESSORIES

Keep accessories light in color, as a scarf or piece of jewelry in the wrong color can overpower you. For your jewelry, beads in your accent colors as well as all shades of pearls (other than black) will look wonderful, especially in lifting a darker-shade top or jacket.

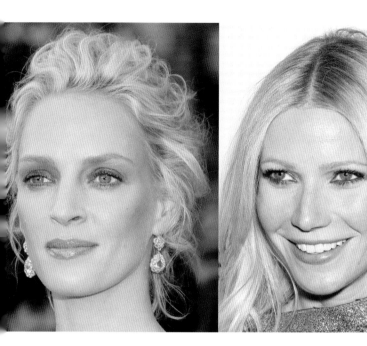
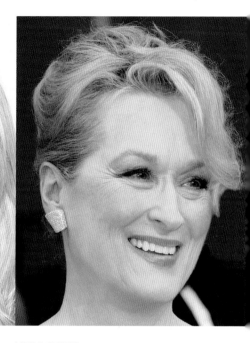

UMA THURMAN

Uma's light, golden blonde hair, blue eyes, and warm skin make her a typical Light with warm undertones.

GWYNETH PALTROW

Gwyneth's ash-toned light blonde hair, rose-toned skin, and light blue eyes give her Light appearance a slight cool undertone.

MERYL STREEP

Like many women, Meryl Streep's coloring has become lighter and more delicate as she's aged.

COLORS FOR YOUR WARDROBE

Below we have listed eight core colors that you can use as a basis for your wardrobe. The neutrals are ideal for investment pieces such as coats, jackets. and trousers. They also make a great alternative to black. Accent colors are where you can make the most of your coloring type by livening up your wardrobe.

NEUTRALS

Medium Grey	Light Navy	Cocoa	Taupe

ACCENTS

Pastel Pink	Geranium	Sky Blue	Apple Green

LIGHT PALETTE

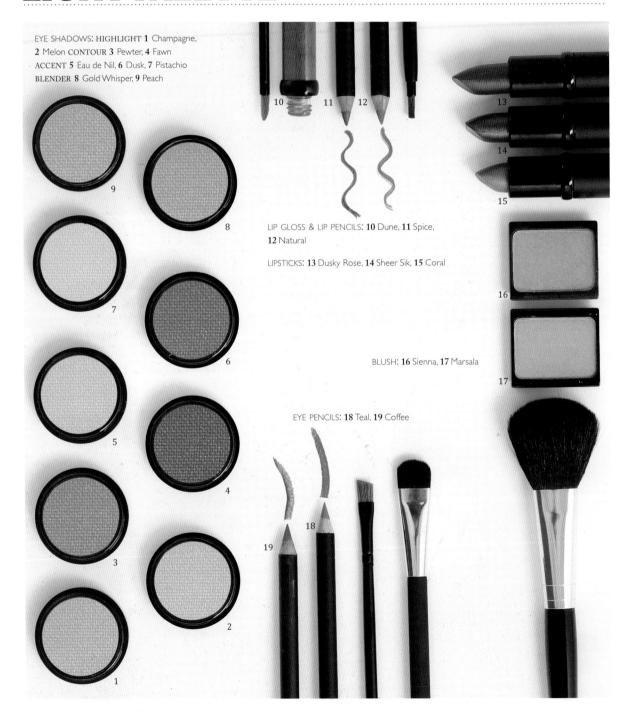

EYE SHADOWS: **HIGHLIGHT 1** Champagne,
2 Melon **CONTOUR 3** Pewter, **4** Fawn
ACCENT 5 Eau de Nil, **6** Dusk, **7** Pistachio
BLENDER 8 Gold Whisper, **9** Peach

LIP GLOSS & LIP PENCILS: **10** Dune, **11** Spice,
12 Natural

LIPSTICKS: **13** Dusky Rose, **14** Sheer Sik, **15** Coral

BLUSH: **16** Sienna, **17** Marsala

EYE PENCILS: **18** Teal, **19** Coffee

A TYPICAL LIGHT

Very light eyebrows

Very light natural blonde hair in either golden or ash tones

Pale green, pale blue, or light brown/ topaz eyes

Porcelain skin, which is often sensitive to the sun and/or skin-care products

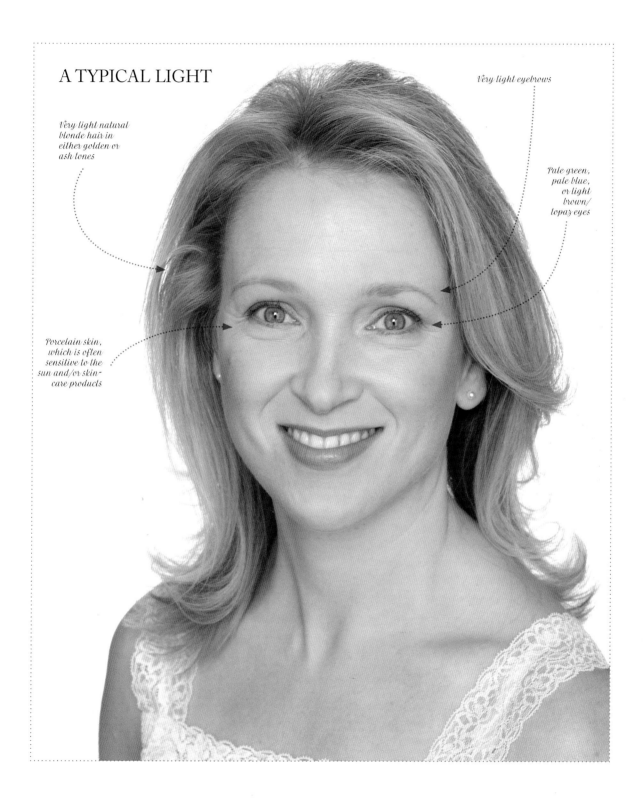

DEEP

Your look is dark and defined, so your make-up should be similarly deep and rich in tone. The key to determining your coloring is that you have dark eyes and hair. Whether you prefer a dramatic look or a natural one, you can create both from the colors in your palette. However, make-up that is too pale, no matter what color your complexion is, can make you look tired.

ARE YOU A DEEP?

Do you have…?

- Dark and defined eyebrows
- Dark eyelashes
- Dark eyes—from dark brown to black
- Medium brown, dark brown, or black hair
- Skin tone in any shade from porcelain to black

MAKE-UP GUIDELINES

- **Face:** To create the perfect canvas, apply a primer to even out your skin tone before your foundation. Choose a foundation that matches your skin tone perfectly. If you like to wear powder, make sure that it tones in with your foundation color. If you have darker skin, there are an increasing number of specialist cosmetic ranges available that offer a wide variety of foundation shades that will work perfectly for you. You may, however, often need to use a mixture of shades to match your skin color.

- **Eyes:** A really dark mascara and eye pencil are essential to enhance the strength of your eye color —you are one of the lucky few coloring types that can pull off black. For a more natural look, go for brown eye pencils. If you want a more dramatic or interesting effect, try aubergine. You have a wonderful array of strong eye shadow colors in your palette; make sure you understand your eye shape (see pages 103–109) to make them up to best effect.

- **Cheeks:** Your blush needs some depth and pigmentation. You might like to use a bronzer instead of a blush, particularly if you have a tan. If you have golden tints to your hair, try a blush with a yellow undertone, such as almond. If your hair has more of a plummy tone, try a blue-based blush such as shiraz.

- **Lips:** To complement your strong look, make sure that your lips are defined. If you prefer not to wear a rich lip color, balance your look with a more dramatic eye make-up. Tomato lipsticks work well with golden or freckled skin, while ruby is great for those with a pinkish tint to their skin. Sheer nutmeg looks great on all the Deeps, regardless of your skin tone.

WEARING COLOR

You have a wonderful range of strong and vibrant colors, including black, that you can wear anytime, day or night. If you are wearing one color on its own, then make sure it is dark or vibrant. In the summer, avoid wearing pale or pastel shades on their own. Either team them up with light colors or go for bolder colors. White can look stunning on you, but dress it up with colorful accessories and dramatic make-up.

ACCESSORIES

Jewelry and other accessories should be strong in color, especially when wearing them with lighter-colored clothes. Pearls and any form of sparkle look stunning against the darker shades from your palette.

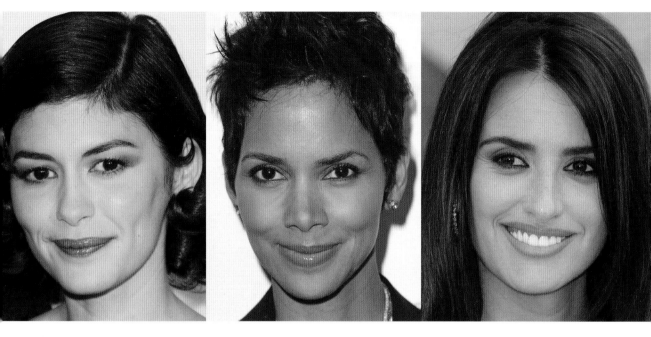

AUDREY TAUTOU

Audrey has cool tones to her skin tone; she should choose dark colors with a cool undertone.

HALLE BERRY

With her black-brown hair and gorgeous brown eyes, Halle has the striking rich look of a Deep. Her make-up colors should be bold to complement her look.

PENELOPE CRUZ

Penelope's deep Mediterranean coloring means she looks best in stronger make-up and clothing colors. Anything that is too pale will wash her out.

COLORS FOR YOUR WARDROBE

Below we have listed eight core colors that you can use as a basis for your wardrobe. The neutrals are ideal for investment pieces such as coats, jackets, and trousers. They also make a great alternative to black. Accent colors are where you can make the most of your coloring type by livening up your wardrobe.

NEUTRALS

Black	Aubergine	Chocolate	Pine

ACCENTS

Royal Purple	Scarlett	Emerald Green	True Blue

DEEP PALETTE

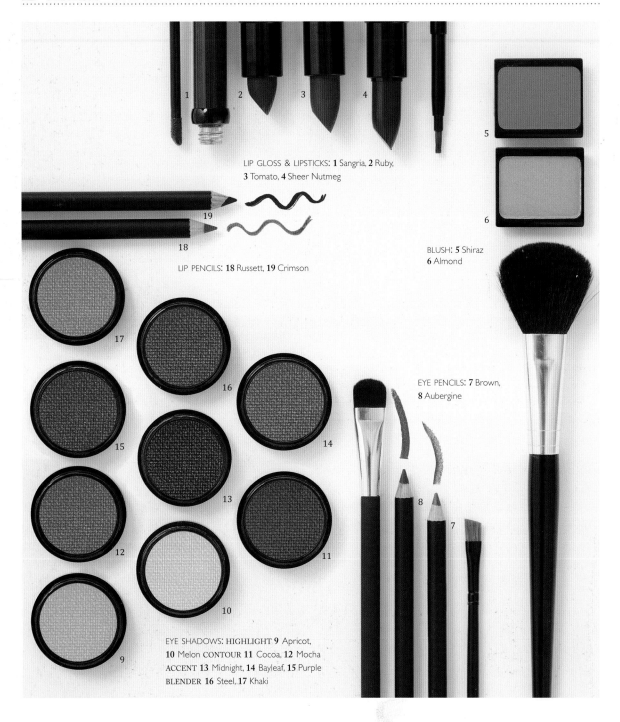

LIP GLOSS & LIPSTICKS: **1** Sangria, **2** Ruby,
3 Tomato, **4** Sheer Nutmeg

LIP PENCILS: **18** Russett, **19** Crimson

BLUSH: **5** Shiraz
6 Almond

EYE PENCILS: **7** Brown,
8 Aubergine

EYE SHADOWS: HIGHLIGHT **9** Apricot,
10 Melon CONTOUR **11** Cocoa, **12** Mocha
ACCENT **13** Midnight, **14** Bayleaf, **15** Purple
BLENDER **16** Steel, **17** Khaki

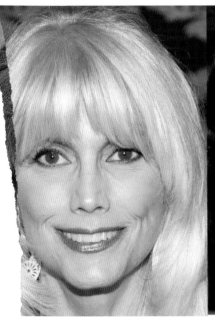 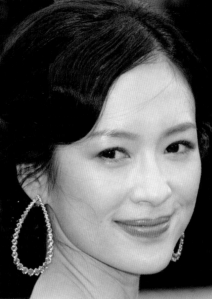 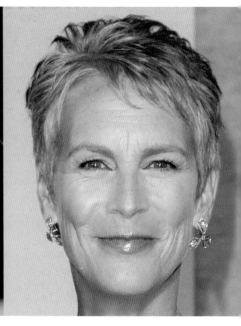

EMMYLOU HARRIS

Emmylou's silver-grey hair, dark eyes, and rose-toned skin make her a typical Cool. She will always look best in blue-based colors.

ZHANG ZIYI

Zhang's absolute porcelain-pale skin with a slight bluish hue and midnight-black hair (with absolutely no warmth to it) make her a beautiful Oriental Cool.

JAMIE LEE CURTIS

Jamie Lee has matured beautifully to a woman with steely grey hair, which gives her a striking Cool look.

COLORS FOR YOUR WARDROBE

Below we have listed eight core colors that you can use as a basis for your wardrobe. The neutrals are ideal for investment pieces such as coats, jackets, and trousers. They also make a great alternative to black. Accent colors are where you can make the most of your coloring type by livening up your wardrobe.

NEUTRALS

| Charcoal | Dark Navy | Spruce | Purple |

ACCENTS

| Light Teal | Rose Pink | Cornflower | Blue Red |

COOL PALETTE

EYE SHADOWS: **HIGHLIGHT 1** Opal,
2 Pearl **CONTOUR 3** Smoke, **4** Pewter
ACCENT 5 Heather, **6** Midnight,
7 Silver Touch **BLENDER 8** Lavender Bliss,
9 Eau de Nil

LIPSTICKS & LIP GLOSS: **10** Bonbon, **11** Ruby,
12 Soft Mauve, **13** Pink Shell

EYE PENCILS: **18** Marine,
19 Amethyst

LIP PENCILS: **14** Rose, **15** Posie

BLUSH: **16** Marsala,
17 Shiraz

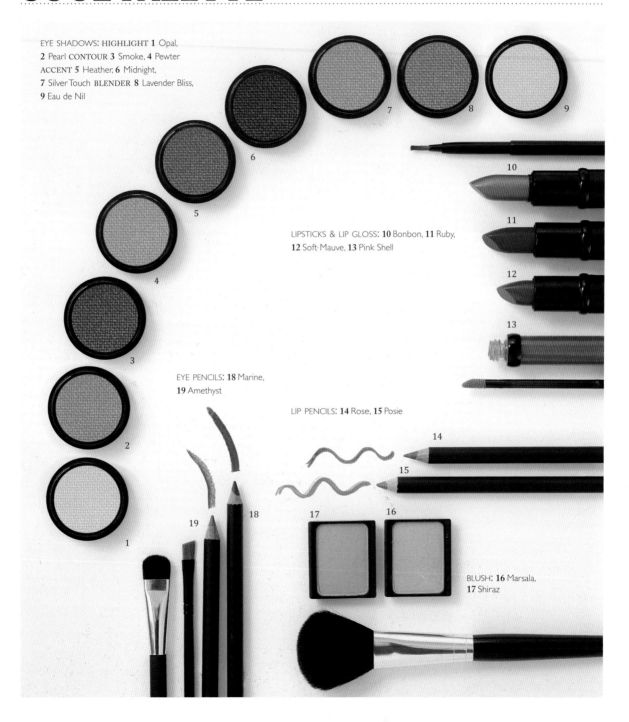

A TYPICAL COOL

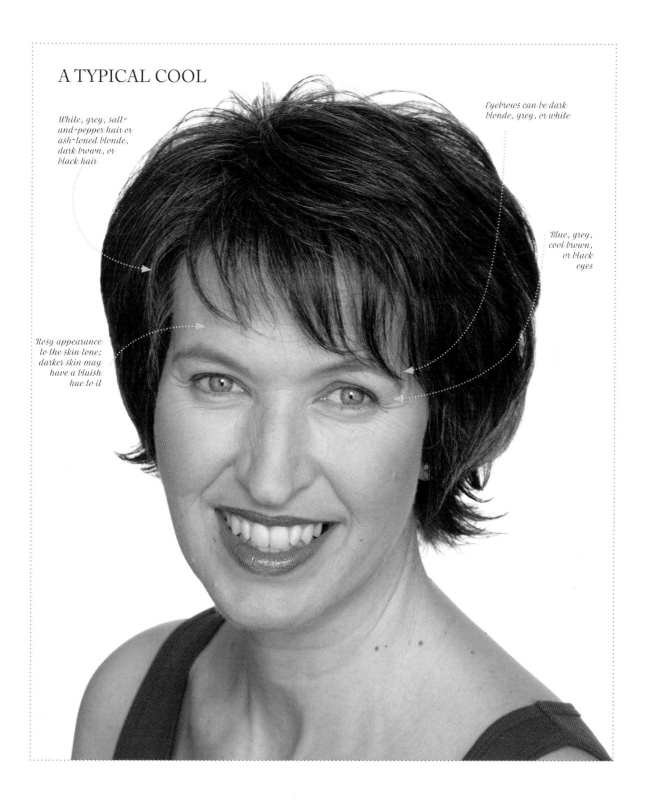

White, grey, salt-and-pepper hair or ash-toned blonde, dark brown, or black hair

Eyebrows can be dark blonde, grey, or white

Blue, grey, cool brown, or black eyes

Rosy appearance to the skin tone; darker skin may have a bluish hue to it

CLEAR

Your most outstanding features are your eyes, which are highlighted because of the contrast to your dark hair. They will have a jewel-like quality to them and sparkle, however you feel. Your eye make-up colors should enhance and not detract from your eye color. As a Clear you can have the choice of making a feature of your eye make-up or your lipstick, but not both.

ARE YOU A CLEAR?

Do you have…?

- Dark eyebrows
- Dark eyelashes
- Clear blue, bright green, or hazel eyes; if you are dark-skinned you will have strong contrast between the whites of your eyes and the iris
- Dark hair
- Skin that can be any tone from light to dark

MAKE-UP GUIDELINES

- **Face:** If you have a porcelain skin, make sure that you choose a foundation color that is not too dark. Embrace your snow-white coloring—it can look fantastic when wearing the right make-up! The key to your look is the contrast between your pale skin and dark hair. Those with darker skin may have dark circles under the eyes, which can detract from your best feature—your eyes. Use a yellow skin primer underneath your eyes to disguise these circles before applying your foundation.

- **Eyes:** Make a feature of your stunning eye color by using colored eye pencils and shadows. If you have blue eyes, try teal eye pencil topped with peppermint eye shadow. Topaz or green eyes will benefit from a hint of silver touch eye shadow. Keep your eyebrows well shaped and defined. To help frame your eyes, use an eyebrow pencil that enhances the rich tones of your natural hair color.

- **Cheeks:** Use your blush to highlight and contour your face, rather than adding color. For those of you with golden hints to your hair, try salmon blush. If you have very dark or black hair, muscat blush will be good for a daytime look. In the summertime, you might want to go for a bronzer or bronzer and blush mixed together.

- **Lips:** Unless you want very dramatic make-up, don't detract from your eyes with a very strong lip color. Using cantaloupe or crimson pencil all over your lips will give any lipstick the clarity it needs to balance with your coloring. As an alternative to lipstick, try just wearing alfresco lip gloss over your favorite color of lip pencil.

WEARING COLOR

Your overall look is to contrast between light and dark shades. If you're wearing one color on its own, it should be a bright one. Avoid tonal looks, especially browns and beiges. If you just can't part with these shades, try wearing them with something bright such as a scarf or a piece of sparkling jewelry. If bright colors frighten you, start to bring them into your wardrobe through patterns, scarves, shoes, and even handbags.

ACCESSORIES

You can go for as many different colors of jewelry as you like—the more glittery and sparkly the better. Diamonds—fake or real—will make a great addition to any outfit.

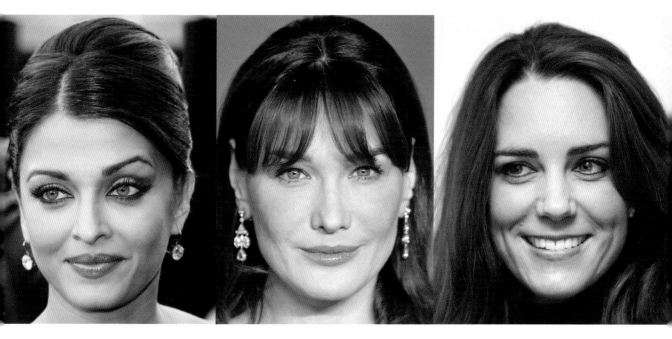

AISHWARYA RAI

The striking contrast between Aishwarya's dark brown hair and piercing green eyes makes her a typical Asian Clear.

CARLA BRUNI

Carla's dark hair really makes her beautiful blue eyes pop—colored eyes are often the first thing that people notice about the Clears.

THE DUCHESS OF CAMBRIDGE

Kate is a typical Clear with her green eyes and dark brown hair. The warmth in her hair and skin tone means that clear colors with a warm undertone suit her best.

COLORS FOR YOUR WARDROBE

Below we have listed eight core colors that you can use as a basis for your wardrobe. The neutrals are ideal for investment pieces such as coats, jackets, and trousers. They also make a great alternative to black. Accent colors are where you can make the most of your coloring type by livening up your wardrobe.

NEUTRALS

ACCENTS

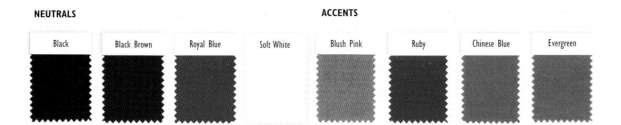

| Black | Black Brown | Royal Blue | Soft White | Blush Pink | Ruby | Chinese Blue | Evergreen |

CLEAR PALETTE

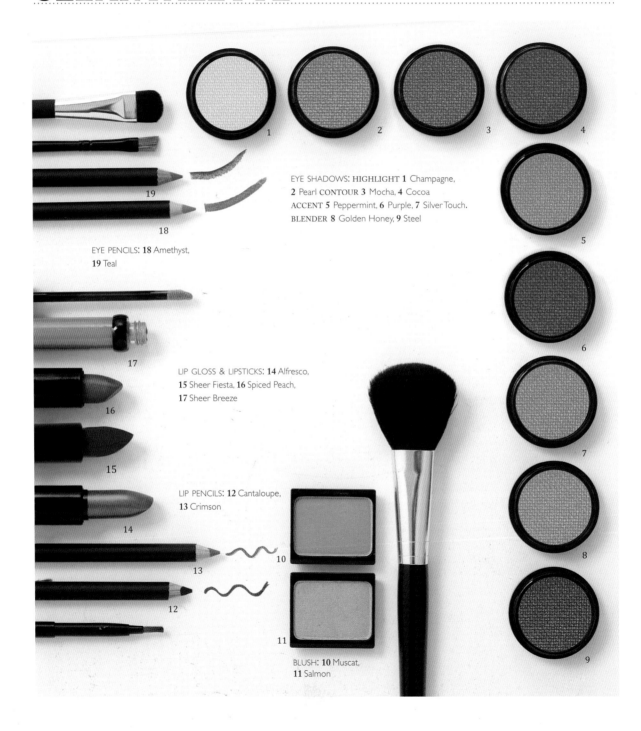

EYE SHADOWS: **HIGHLIGHT 1** Champagne,
2 Pearl **CONTOUR 3** Mocha, **4** Cocoa
ACCENT 5 Peppermint, **6** Purple, **7** Silver Touch.
BLENDER 8 Golden Honey, **9** Steel

EYE PENCILS: **18** Amethyst,
19 Teal

LIP GLOSS & LIPSTICKS: **14** Alfresco,
15 Sheer Fiesta, **16** Spiced Peach,
17 Sheer Breeze

LIP PENCILS: **12** Cantaloupe,
13 Crimson

BLUSH: **10** Muscat,
11 Salmon

A TYPICAL CLEAR

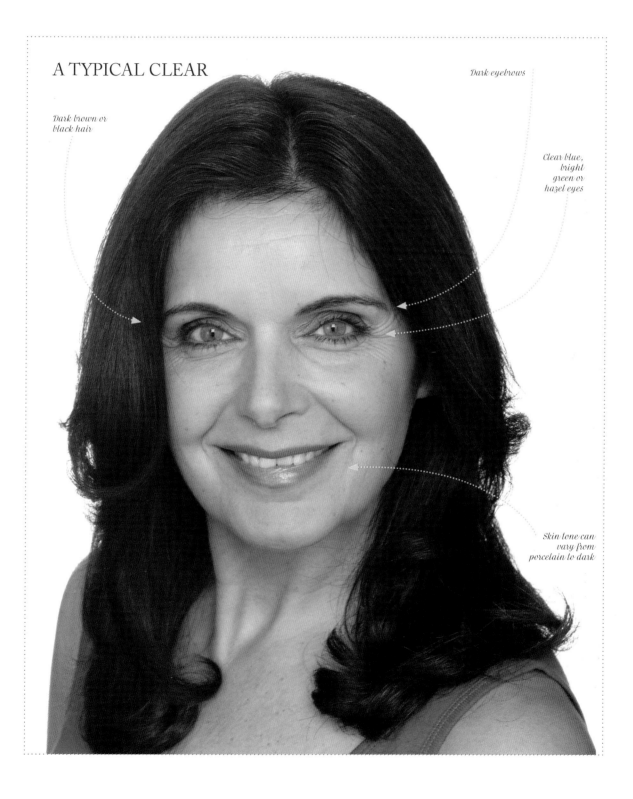

Dark brown or black hair

Dark eyebrows

Clear blue, bright green or hazel eyes

Skin tone can vary from porcelain to dark

SOFT

You may have found a little of yourself in each of the previous coloring types, but did not fit exactly. The gentle combination of your hair, skin, and eye color means that your make-up needs to be soft and subtle. That doesn't mean that you don't need to apply your make-up every day. Leaving the house without your lipstick is not an option—you need color and definition.

ARE YOU A SOFT?

Do you have…?

- Blonde to dark brown eyebrows
- Blonde to dark brown eyelashes
- Soft blue, soft green, soft shades of hazel or brown eyes; your eyes will often change color depending on your mood and what you wear
- Mousy blonde to light brown hair, often with highlights
- Medium depth of skin tone

MAKE-UP GUIDELINES

- **Face:** Because of your medium-depth skin tone, you may find it easier to blend two shades of foundation together to get the perfect match. That way, in the summer when you have a slight tan, you can use the darker shade and in winter, when you are paler, you can just use the lighter one. Remember to even out pinkness or discoloration with a skin primer or skin adjuster before applying your foundation.
- **Eyes:** Don't overpower the subtle shades of your eyes with strong, vibrant eye shadow colors and pencils; instead use golds, smoky greys, and soft greens. Go for a black brown mascara, which is softer and more flattering than black. Blue-grey eyes will look great with granite eye pencil, whereas moss eye pencil will flatter brown or hazel eyes. Make sure you blend all shades of your eye shadows together well.
- **Cheeks:** When applying blush, make sure you really blend it in to complement your subtle look. Candy blush works well if you have more of a rosy skin tone, whereas sienna is a great blush if you have a more yellow/warm undertone to your skin.
- **Lips:** Always use a lip pencil to define your lips and be careful not to overpower your look with strong lip colors. Lip glosses are a great alternative to lipsticks for the Softs, as they are more subtle. Try a warm sand lip gloss worn over natural or spice lip pencil.

WEARING COLOR

Tone-on-tone color combinations are your best look. This can be achieved by choosing colours from the same color family, for example different shades of taupes and browns or light navy and charcoal blue worn together. Keep away from anything too vibrant, as it will not balance with your coloring. Black will be too overpowering for you, particularly near your face, so try substituting charcoal instead. If you still want a little black dress, try it in black lace or chiffon, which are softer than a shiny black satin, for example.

ACCESSORIES

Keep jewelry colors blended and not too shiny. Matte metals are best, and stones of any color work well. Jewelry made of natural materials, such as wood, leather or fabrics, is also wonderful. Bring in accent colors with scarves or bags.

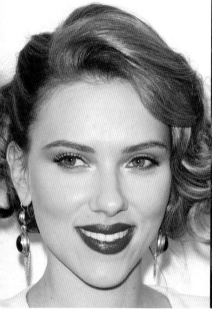

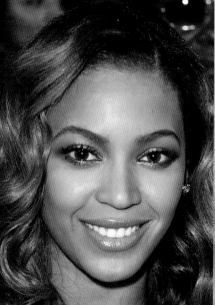

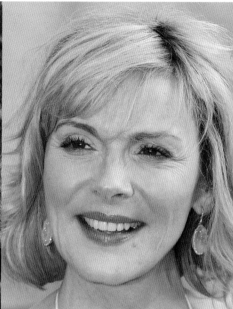

SCARLETT JOHANSSON

Scarlett's blonde hair, dark green eyes, and fair skin tone all have a bit of warmth to them, meaning soft colors with yellow undertones will suit her.

BEYONCÉ

Beyoncé's dark blonde highlights blend subtly with her skin tone and eye color, giving her an overall softer look.

KIM CATTRALL

Many maturing women, like Kim Cattrall, choose to highlight or lighten their hair and find it a more flattering, softer look as they age.

COLORS FOR YOUR WARDROBE

Below we have listed eight core colors that you can use as a basis for your wardrobe. The neutrals are ideal for investment pieces such as coats, jackets, and trousers. They also make a great alternative to black. Accent colors are where you can make the most of your coloring type by livening up your wardrobe.

NEUTRALS

Rose Brown	Charcoal	Charcoal Blue	Stone

ACCENTS

Claret	Sage	Soft Violet	Light Perwinkle

SOFT PALETTE

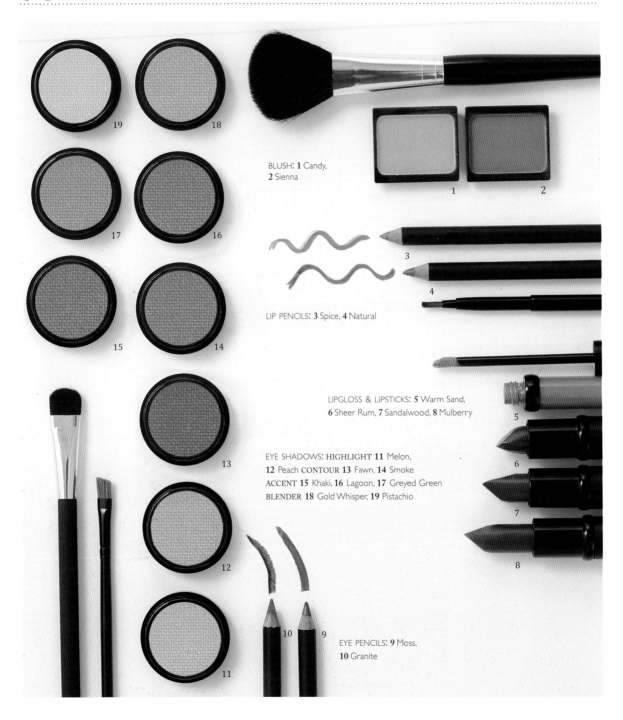

BLUSH: **1** Candy,
2 Sienna

LIP PENCILS: **3** Spice, **4** Natural

LIPGLOSS & LIPSTICKS: **5** Warm Sand,
6 Sheer Rum, **7** Sandalwood, **8** Mulberry

EYE SHADOWS: HIGHLIGHT **11** Melon,
12 Peach CONTOUR **13** Fawn, **14** Smoke
ACCENT **15** Khaki, **16** Lagoon, **17** Greyed Green
BLENDER **18** Gold Whisper, **19** Pistachio

EYE PENCILS: **9** Moss,
10 Granite

A TYPICAL SOFT

Light brown, mousy blonde, or blonde hair, often with highlights

Blonde to dark brown eyebrows

Medium blue, green, hazel, or brown eyes

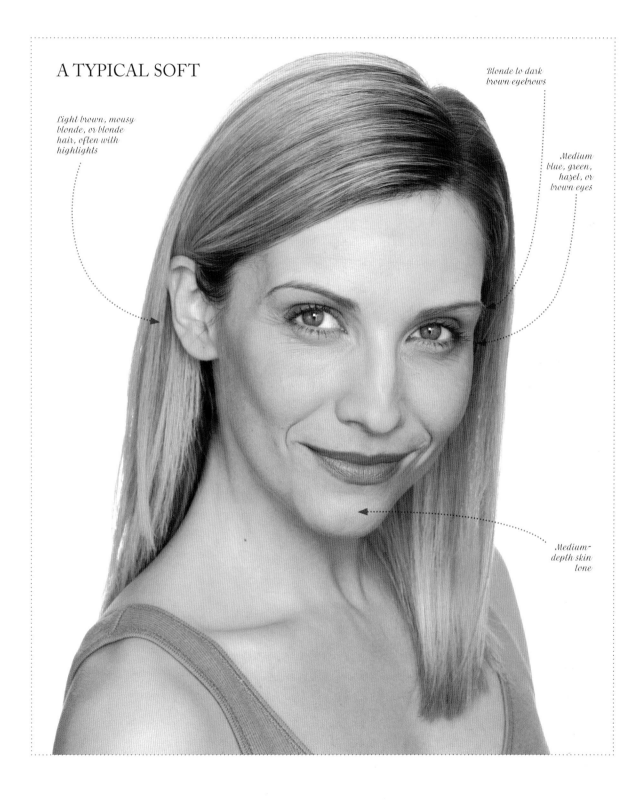

Medium-depth skin tone

DIFFERENT
LOOKS

Now that you're familiar with your coloring, the make-up that works for you, and how to apply it, you can achieve a range of key looks. Using a "barely-there" base as your starting point, you can build on this to a made-up daytime look, developing it further into an evening look, and finally to a full-on glamour look for those special occasions. All of the looks develop from preparing your face—using primer, foundation, or tinted moisturizer and powder. Unless otherwise stated, apply fresh lipstick for each key look.

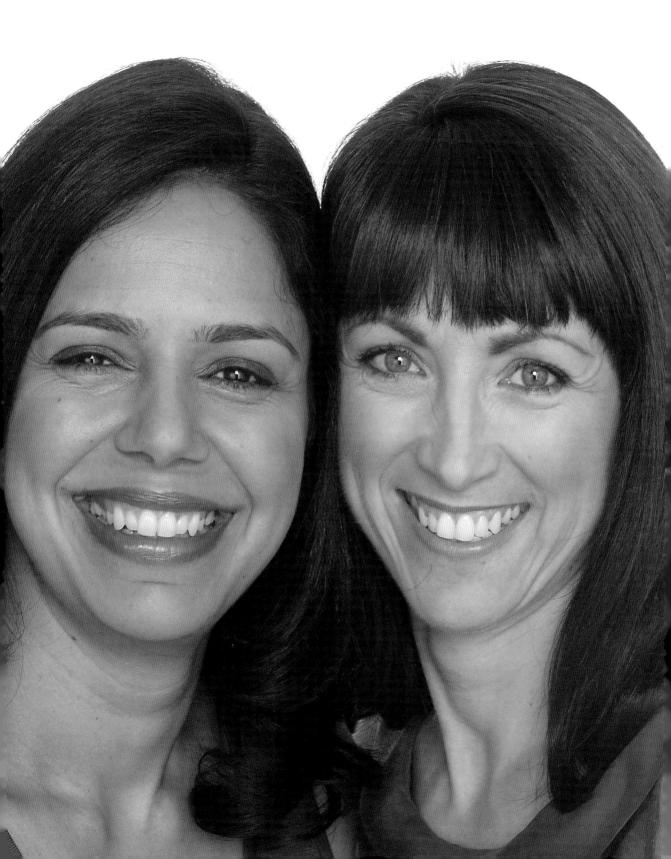

LIGHT: FOUR KEY LOOKS

When it comes to different make-up looks, it's all about adding subtle definition to your Light features. Give a hint of color to eyebrows and eyelashes—a warm brown mascara will be more flattering than black.

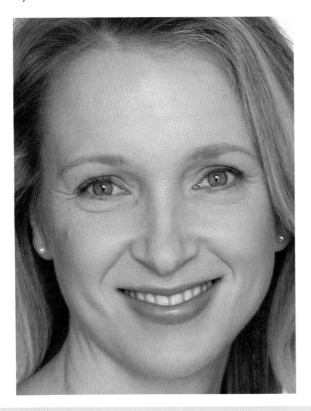 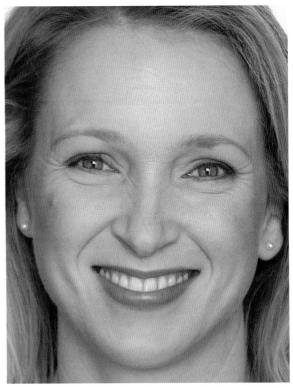

YOU WILL NEED Coffee eye pencil, Champagne eye shadow, Blonde eyebrow pencil, Warm brown mascara, Marsala blush, Spice lip pencil, Coral lipstick

YOU WILL NEED Pewter eye shadow, Coffee eye pencil, Marsala blush, Spice lip pencil, Coral lipstick, Dune lip gloss

Barely there (base)

Apply coffee eye pencil along top and bottom lash lines, then blend champagne eye shadow all over the eye area. Define the brows with blonde eyebrow pencil. Use warm brown mascara to give your lashes some life. Add a touch of marsala blush to the cheeks, then use spice lip pencil all over the lips and lightly apply coral lipstick over the top.

Daytime (apply over Barelythere)

Apply pewter eye shadow on the eyelid only, then redefine the lash lines with a little more coffee eye pencil. Add a little more marsala blush to the cheeks. Reapply spice lip pencil and coral lipstick, finally topping with dune lip gloss.

Try not to overpower your delicate coloring with strong shades of eye shadow or lipstick, even when it comes to more glamorous make-up. Instead, use the right colors from your palette and apply them in different ways.

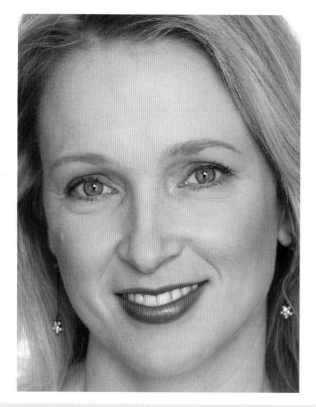

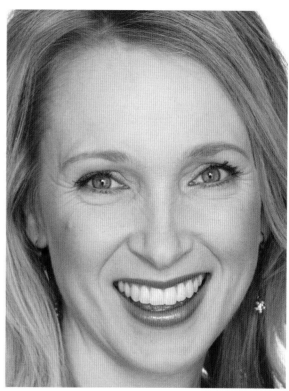

YOU WILL NEED Teal eye pencil, Dusk eye shadow, Champagne eye shadow, Blonde eyebrow pencil, Iridescent highlighter, Sienna blush, Natural lip pencil, Sheer silk lipstick

YOU WILL NEED Teal eye pencil, Pistachio eye shadow, Sienna blush, Coral lipstick, Dune lip gloss

Casual Evening (apply over Daytime)

Apply teal pencil along top and bottom lash lines over coffee; blend into the outer corners. Brush dusk eye shadow over the eyelids; blend into the sockets. Highlight the brow bone with champagne shadow; redefine brows with more blonde pencil. Add highlighter along cheekbones and blend with sienna blush. Use natural lip pencil all over lips; finish with sheer silk lipstick.

Night Glamour (apply over Casual Evening)

Thicken the teal pencil along top and bottom lash lines and blend well into the outer corners of the eyes. Apply pistachio eye shadow all over the eyelids. Add some more sienna blush to the cheeks. Use coral lipstick all over the lips, and finally, add dune lip gloss.

DEEP: FOUR KEY LOOKS

You are lucky that your stunning features have a lot of depth to them and stand out on their own. Accentuate your look by complementing it with dark, rich colors, even when it comes to more subtle daytime looks.

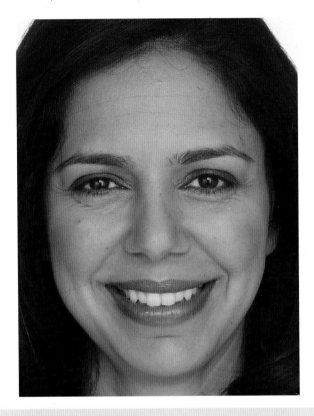

YOU WILL NEED Brown eye pencil, Cocoa eye shadow, Apricot eye shadow, Black brown mascara, Almond blush, Sangria lip gloss

YOU WILL NEED Brown eye pencil, Cocoa eye shadow, Mocha eye shadow, Apricot eye shadow, Shiraz blush, Russet lip pencil, Sheer Nutmeg lipstick

Barely there (base)

Use the brown eye pencil along top and bottom lash lines. Apply cocoa eye shadow all over the eyelids and blend well with apricot eye shadow along the brow bone to highlight the eye. Use black brown mascara to add depth to your eye lashes. Apply almond blush to the cheeks very lightly. Use sangria lip gloss on the lips.

Daytime (apply over Barely there)

Thicken the lash lines with more brown eye pencil and add a bit more cocoa eye shadow all over the lids. Use mocha eye shadow to blend into the corners. Add more apricot eye shadow to highlight the brow bone. Apply shiraz blush to the cheeks. Apply russet lip pencil all over the lips and then top with sheer nutmeg lipstick.

Blushers will need some depth to balance out your coloring. Lipsticks in rich shades will look fantastic on you; however, if you prefer softer colors you will need to ensure that your face is balanced with strong eye make-up.

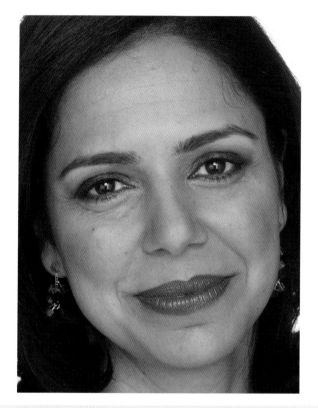

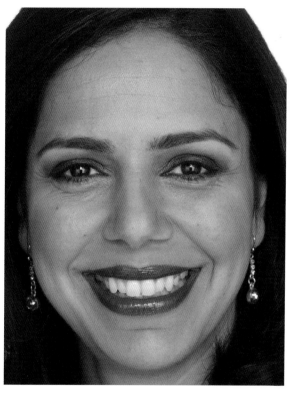

YOU WILL NEED Aubergine eye pencil, Khaki eye shadow, Bayleaf eye shadow, Shiraz blush, Russet lip pencil, Tomato lipstick

YOU WILL NEED Aubergine eye pencil, Melon eye shadow, Midnight eye shadow, Shiraz blush, Crimson lip pencil, Ruby lipstick, Sangria lip gloss

Casual Evening *(apply over Daytime)*

Apply aubergine pencil along the lash line quite strongly. Use khaki eye shadow all over the lid and then blend bayleaf eye shadow well into the corners of the eye. Define the shiraz blush a little more. Use russet lip pencil all over the lips and top with tomato lipstick.

Night Glamour *(apply over Casual Evening)*

Apply aubergine eye pencil along the top and bottom lash lines. Highlight the brow bone with melon eye shadow. Apply midnight eye shadow all over the eyelids and blend over the upper and bottom lash lines. Use shiraz blush to give definition to the cheeks. Line and fill the lips with crimson lip pencil, followed by ruby lipstick and sangria lip gloss.

WARM: FOUR KEY LOOKS

To enhance your warm and rich coloring, your make-up should always have yellow undertones. Brown eye pencils and mascara flatter more than black for both day and night. Choose a blush powder with a warm undertone

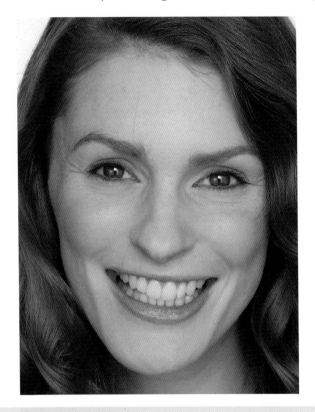

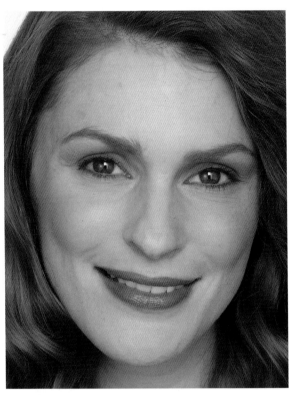

YOU WILL NEED Peach eye shadow, Brown eye pencil, Muscat blush, Warm brown mascara, Warm Sand lip gloss

YOU WILL NEED Cocoa eye shadow, Peach eye shadow, Moss eye pencil, Khaki eye shadow, Spice lip pencil, Terracotta lipstick

Barely there (base)

Apply peach eye shadow all over the eyelids; add brown eye pencil very thinly along the top and bottom lash lines. Add a touch of muscat blush to top of the cheekbones. Apply warm brown mascara to top lashes only. Add some color to the lips with warm sand lip gloss.

Daytime (apply over Barely there)

Add cocoa eye shadow all over the eyelids and apply more peach eye shadow to highlight the brow bone. Apply moss pencil on top of the brown eye pencil, adding depth to the outer corners. Define the eyes by adding khaki eye shadow to the outer corners and along the pencil line. Use spice lip pencil all over the lips and finish with terracotta lipstick.

and simply apply with a bit more depth depending on the time of day or occasion. Whether you want subtle lip color or more dramatic lips, keep your lip color warm with lovely, golden earthy tones.

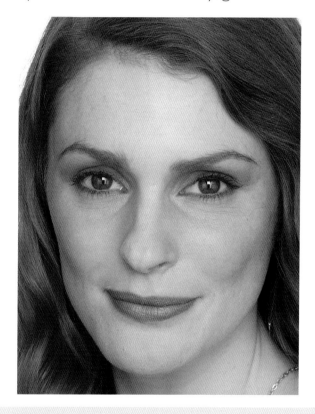

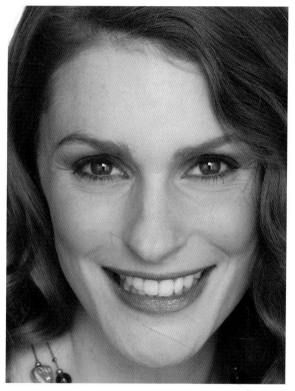

YOU WILL NEED Khaki eye shadow, Moss eye pencil, Greyed Green eye shadow, Salmon blush, Brown black mascara, Cantaloupe lip pencil, Warm Pink lipstick

YOU WILL NEED Brown eye pencil, Fawn eye shadow, Peach eye shadow, Iridescent highlighter, Brown black mascara, Spice lip pencil, Sheer Copper lipstick

Casual Evening *(apply over Daytime)*

Apply khaki eye shadow all over the eyelids; deepen the moss eye pencil, concentrating it on the outer edges. Add some greyed green eye shadow to the center of each eye. Apply a darker shade of mascara, such as brown black. Use salmon blush to give definition to the cheekbones. Add cantaloupe lip pencil all over and finish with warm pink lipstick.

Night Glamour *(apply over Casual Evening)*

Use brown eye pencil over the top and bottom lash lines. Apply fawn eye shadow over the entire eyelid and add more peach eye shadow to the brow bone. Use iridescent highlighter along the cheekbones. Redefine the lashes with another coat of brown black mascara. Cover the lips with spice lip pencil and then apply sheer copper lipstick all over.

COOL: FOUR KEY LOOKS

Cool, blue-based tones of eye shadows, blush, and lipstick will always look best on you, regardless of what look you are trying to achieve. Use a pink blush powder to define your cheekbones. Take your barely-there make-up

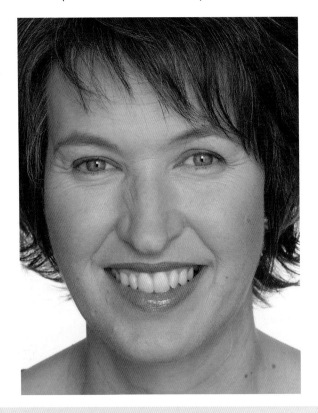 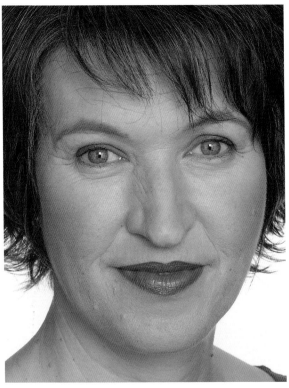

YOU WILL NEED Pewter eye shadow, Marine eye pencil, Blonde eyebrow pencil, Navy mascara, Marsala blush, Pink Shell lip gloss

YOU WILL NEED Marine eye pencil, Heather eye shadow, Silver Touch eye shadow, Opal eye shadow, Marsala blush, Posie lip pencil, Pink Shell lip gloss

Barely there (base)

Apply pewter eye shadow all over the eyelids, followed by marine eye pencil along the top and bottom lash lines, blending in well. Define the brows with blonde eyebrow pencil. Apply navy mascara on the top and bottom lashes. Add a touch of marsala blush on the cheeks, and finish with pink shell lip gloss.

Daytime (apply over Barely there)

Redefine the eye line with marine eye pencil, both top and bottom, blending well into the outer corners. Apply heather eye shadow all over the lids and silver touch eye shadow blended into the corners. Apply opal eye shadow on the brow bone to highlight it. Reapply marsala blush. Use posie lip pencil all over the lips and top with pink shell lip gloss.

up a notch by defining the eye area, and do so more and more, with grey, blue, and lilac shades of eye shadows and eye pencils. Lips will look great in a soft pink gloss for the daytime or bold ruby reds for instant glamour.

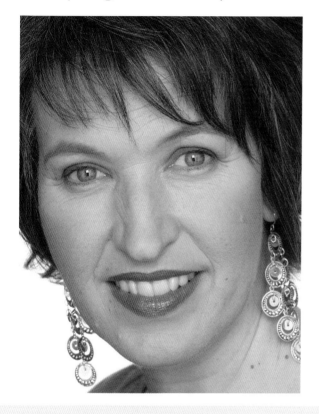

YOU WILL NEED Smoke eye shadow, Amethyst eye pencil, Opal eye shadow, Iridescent highlighter, Ruby lipstick, Pink Shell lip gloss

YOU WILL NEED Midnight eye shadow, Marine eye pencil, Shiraz blush, Rose lip pencil, Soft Mauve lipstick, Pink Shell lip gloss

Casual Evening *(apply over Daytime)*

Apply smoke eye shadow all over the eyelids. Use amethyst eye pencil fairly thickly on the lash line, top and bottom, and blend in. Highlight the brow bone with opal eye shadow and use the iridescent highlighter on the top of the cheekbones. Apply ruby lipstick, topped off with pink shell lip gloss.

Night Glamour *(apply over Casual Evening)*

Apply midnight eye shadow to the outer corners of the eyes and the sockets. Intensify the eye pencil with marine along the top and bottom lash lines, blending well. Apply shiraz blush. Use rose lip pencil all over the lips, topping with soft mauve lipstick and pink shell lip gloss.

CLEAR: FOUR KEY LOOKS

Whatever your make-up look, it is all about making the most of your best feature—your fabulous eyes. Forget the rules about matching your eye shadow to your eye color—it will only make your eyes blend in with your

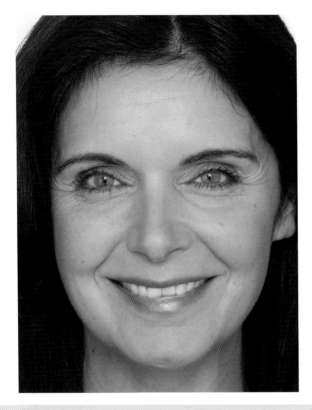
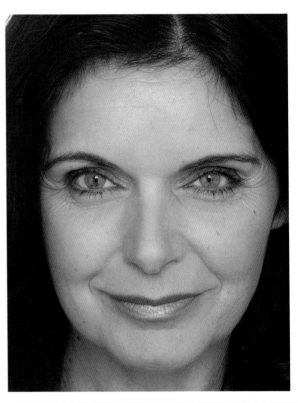

YOU WILL NEED Champagne eye shadow, Teal eye pencil, Black brown mascara, Muscat blush, Sheer Breeze lipstick

YOU WILL NEED Teal eye pencil, Peppermint eye shadow, Pearl eye shadow, Muscat blush, Sheer Breeze lipstick, Cantaloupe lip pencil, Alfresco lip gloss

Barely there (base)

Use champagne eye shadow all over the eye area, and then apply teal eye pencil along the lash lines, top and bottom. Use a black brown mascara on the top and bottom lashes. Apply a touch of muscat blush to the cheeks. Use sheer breeze lipstick.

Daytime (apply over Barely there)

Reapply an additional layer of teal eye pencil, then add peppermint eye shadow all over the eyelids up to the socket lines. Add pearl shadow to the center of the lids and blend in. Add a little more muscat blush to the cheeks. Define sheer breeze lipstick with cantaloupe lip pencil, topping off with alfresco lip gloss.

look, and you really should make them pop. Bright colors, such as teal pencil with peppermint eye shadow, are great during the day, whereas aubergine pencil and purple eye shadows will be more glamorous for the evening.

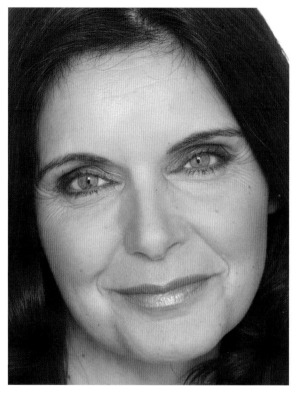

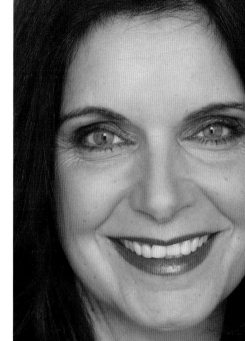

YOU WILL NEED Mocha eye shadow, Amethyst eye pencil, Salmon blush, Cantaloupe lip pencil, Spiced Peach lipstick, Alfresco lip gloss

YOU WILL NEED Purple eye shadow, Amethyst eye pencil, Blonde eyebrow pencil, Iridescent highlighter, Crimson lip pencil, Sheer Fiesta lipstick

Casual Evening (apply over Daytime)

Apply mocha eye shadow over the eyelids, blending well into the outer corners of the eye. Apply amethyst eye pencil over the teal. Blend salmon blush with the already applied muscat. Now use cantaloupe lip pencil all over the lips, adding spiced peach lipstick and finishing with alfresco lip gloss.

Night Glamour (apply over Casual Evening)

For greater definition, apply purple eye shadow all over the eyelids and add more amethyst eye pencil on top and bottom lash lines. Define the eyebrows well using blonde eyebrow pencil. Apply iridescent highlighter in a "C" shape along the brow bone and to the top of cheekbones. Use crimson lip pencil to define the lips and top with sheer fiesta lipstick.

SOFT: FOUR KEY LOOKS

Your soft coloring needs to be complemented with muted tones. Anything that is too bright or dark will detract from your lovely face. Your eyebrows should always be defined with a blonde eyebrow pencil, while your eyes

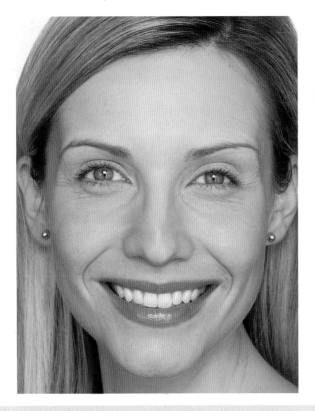 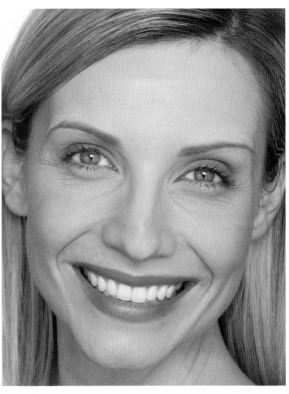

YOU WILL NEED Melon eye shadow, Warm brown mascara, Blonde eyebrow pencil, Sienna blush, Warm Sand lip gloss

YOU WILL NEED Fawn eye shadow, Gold Whisper eye shadow, Moss eye pencil, Sienna blush, Natural lip pencil, Sandalwood lipstick

Barely there (base)

Add a wash of melon eye shadow all over the eye area, add a touch of warm brown mascara to give definition to lashes. Apply blonde eyebrow pencil to the eyebrows. Add a touch of sienna blush to the cheeks. Warm sand lip gloss will give a lovely light gloss to the lips.

Daytime (apply over Barely there)

Apply fawn eye shadow all over lid and then add gold whisper to the brow area. Apply moss eye pencil along the top and bottom lash line and blend well into the outer corners. Define blush with another application of sienna. Use natural lip pencil all over and finish with sandalwood lipstick.

need to be lined with soft browns or moss shades, not black. Natural, subtle lip shades are perfect for daytime; for an evening out, go for softer colors with a little more pigment, topped with a subtle gloss for a lovely sheen.

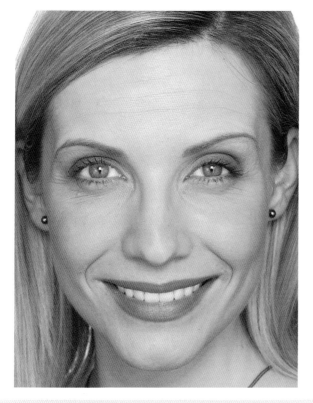

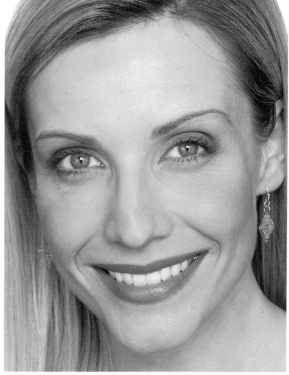

YOU WILL NEED Smoke eye shadow, Gold Whisper eye shadow, Granite eye pencil, Candy blush, Spice lip pencil, Sheer Rum lipstick Warm Sand lip gloss

YOU WILL NEED Gold Whisper eye shadow, Granite eye pencil, Iridescent highlighter, Natural lip pencil, Mulberry lipstick, Warm Sand lip gloss

Casual Evening (apply over Daytime)

Apply smoke eye shadow to the outer corner and up into the socket lines and blend in. Add a little gold whisper eye shadow as a highlighter to the brow bone. Apply granite eye pencil along the upper and lower lash lines. Add candy blush on the cheeks. Use spice lip pencil all over lips, followed by sheer rum lipstick, then warm sand lip gloss to finish.

Night Glamour (apply over Casual Evening)

Add gold whisper eye shadow to the eyelids. Redefine the eye lines with another application of granite eye pencil. Use iridescent highlighter along the top of the cheekbones to give a glamorous look without being too heavy. Use the natural lip pencil all over the lips, then follow with mulberry lipstick and top with warm sand lip gloss.

AGE-PROOF
YOUR MAKE-UP

It is easy to get stuck in a skincare and make-up rut, wearing your make-up the way you were first taught—and often using the same make-up that you've come to know and love, year after year. However, the colors you wear and the way you apply your make-up in your twenties may not be suitable as you mature. Simply adapting your skincare routine and wearing age-appropriate make-up will improve the appearance of your skin and disguise minor signs of aging, as well as make you look and feel younger.

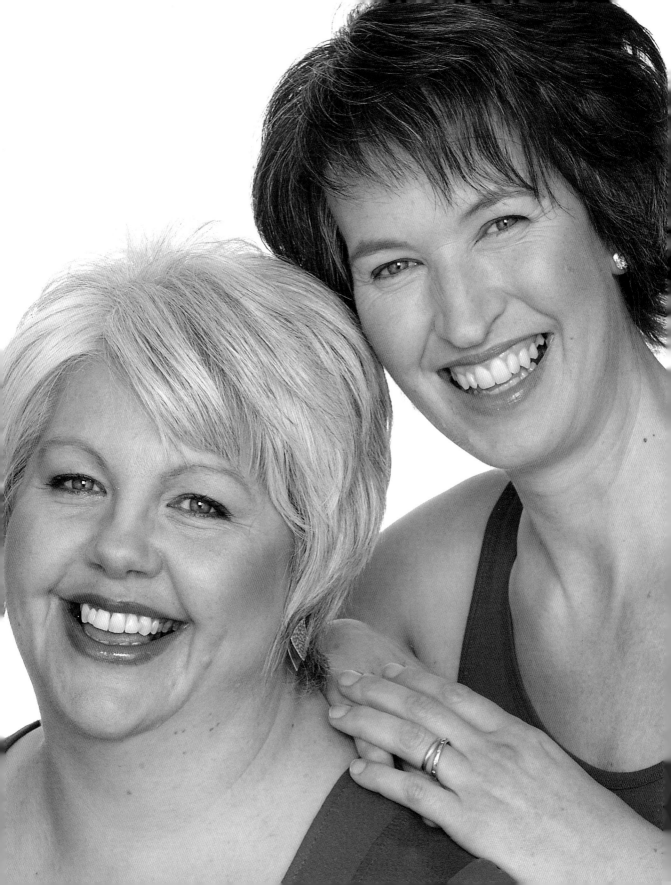

IN YOUR THIRTIES

This is the age when most women begin to see the first signs of aging— perhaps fine lines around the eyes and slightly deeper lines around the nose and mouth. If you haven't been using night and eye creams, now is the time to start. To help counter the effects of aging, it is also a good time to start doing facial workout exercises—see pages 24–25.

If you are beginning to notice the signs of aging, take a trip to an established skincare counter and look at the latest products that are available, as the science of skincare is changing constantly. The earlier you start to use skincare products, the less the signs of aging will show in the long term.

MAKE-UP

In your twenties you may have been lucky enough not to have to wear very much make-up, if any at all. However, in your thirties there may be some discoloration of your skin due to sun damage or hormonal changes after childbirth. Now is the time to start to use some basic make-up techniques to keep you looking well groomed at all times.

KEY POINTS

- Shape your eyebrows regularly.
- Use a skin primer to even out your skin tone.
- Choose foundation to match your skin color.
- Define your eyes with eye pencil.
- Use appropriate colors for your coloring type (see Chapter 3, pages 48–75).
- Use your blush to contour the face.
- Iridescent highlighters are great to define your bone structure.
- Lip pencils, lipsticks, and lip glosses will add color and a sense of fashion to your look.

COMMON PITFALLS

Avoid falling into the trap of buying high-fashion colors just because your favorite magazine tells you that this is this season's look. In your teens and twenties, you can play with fashion make-up and wearing the right colors for your coloring isn't as important. However, when you're in your thirties, you should start to individualize your own look, rather than wearing the same colors and trends as all your friends. A daytime lipstick will give you an instant lift, and mascara is a basic essential to define your eyes.

SKINCARE ROUTINES FOR YOUR THIRTIES

Daily

- Cleanse and tone twice a day.
- Moisturize in the morning and use an eye gel.
- Nourish with night cream and eye cream before you go to bed.

Weekly

- Exfoliate your face twice a week.
- If you are still suffering from slightly oily skin and open pores, use a clay-type mask once a week after steaming your face.

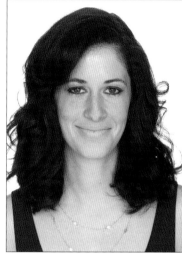

TRY TO AVOID…

An unbalanced look with heavy eye make-up, no foundation, and pale lips.

GET THE RIGHT LOOK

Use a foundation to even out skin tone. Complete the look by using eye make-up in your correct colors and balance the face with defined color on the lips. Add a hint of color with blush to give definition to your facial features.

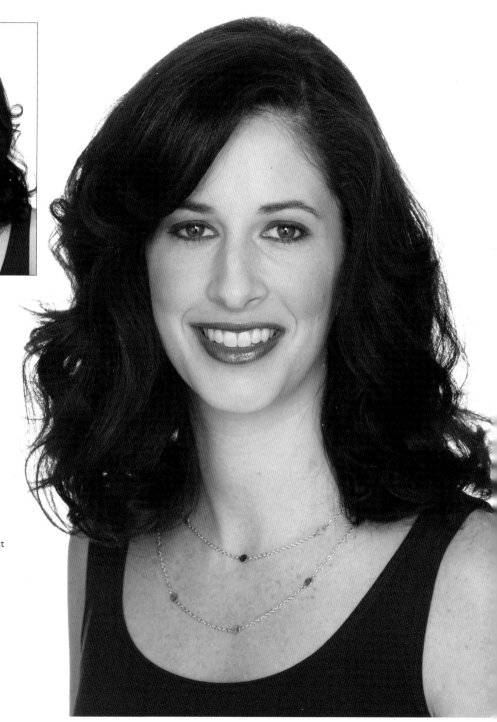

IN YOUR FORTIES

By now you will have established a regular skincare routine. You may see more lines appearing on your face and your eyelids may start to become a little crêpey. These signs of aging will depend on your genetics; if your mother kept a youthful look, you will probably have inherited her genes. Be sure to keep your make-up natural, and adapt it to your changing skin.

MAKE-UP

Now is the time to turn your make-up into something that is sophisticated but still easy to apply, as you will probably have a busy lifestyle. Make-up can also be used to hide imperfections on your skin. Your make-up still needs to look natural, but that might take a little more care and attention.

KEY POINTS

- An eyebrow pencil may be a great addition to your make-up bag, to give your brows definition.
- Consider tinting your eyelashes, which will give extra definition alongside your mascara.
- Shimmer on your eyes will still look great—but avoid very sparkly fashion shades.
- Use a light concealer (rather than a heavy, creamy, stick type) to disguise dark circles under the eyes.
- Apply eye pencil two-thirds on the top and halfway underneath. Try to use colors other than black.
- Apply your blush along the top of your cheekbones, which is very flattering, rather than the hollows.
- Give your lips more definition by layering your lip colors, starting with lip pencil, then lipstick, and finishing off with a gloss.

COMMON PITFALLS

Some fashion products, such as the heavy false eyelashes, iridescent highlighters, shimmer sticks, and fake tans you used in your thirties during the day, should now be kept for your glamour and evening looks. Your skin may not be as even toned as it once was, so try a primer to balance out the different areas. Also, tinted moisturizers may not give you enough coverage, so you should start to consider a heavier liquid foundation. A proper skincare routine is now essential—especially moisturizing at night.

SKINCARE ROUTINES FOR YOUR FORTIES

Daily

- Cleanse and tone twice a day with a lotion or cream cleanser.
- Moisturize in the morning and use an eye gel.
- Nourish with night cream and eye cream before you go to bed.
- Start using a skin serum that will encourage cell renewal, which slows down the signs of aging.

Weekly

- Exfoliate your face twice a week.
- Use a firming, moisturizing mask once a week; on open pores, use a clay-type mask once a week after steaming your face.

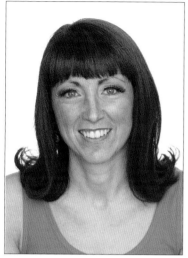

TRY TO AVOID…

Too much fake tan, which has an aging effect. Now's the time to also give up false eyelashes and frosty lipsticks.

GET THE RIGHT LOOK

A little more attention is required to give you a sophisticated look for your forties. Make-up colors should be slightly softened for a natural daytime look—for example, choose black brown mascara rather than black. If you are prone to dark circles under the eyes, a skin primer or light concealer can help brighten up your eyes.

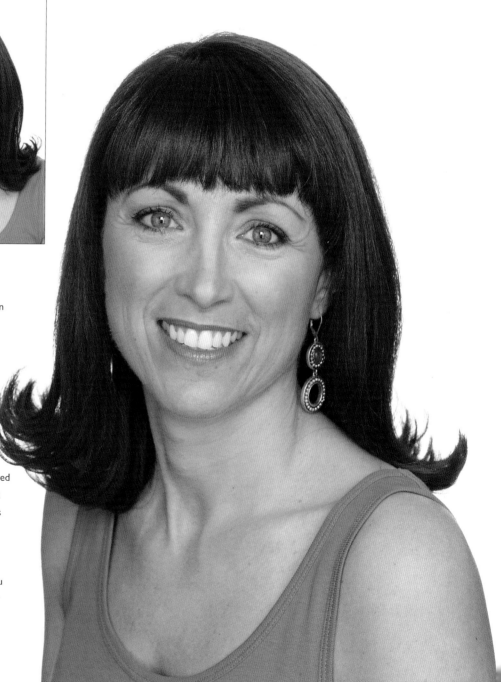

IN YOUR FIFTIES

Your fifties is the decade when nature interferes with your skincare routine and can result in changes to the muscle tone and texture on your face, which is all down to hormones. However, carrying a little extra weight can act as natural Botox. With a balanced diet, exercise, good skincare, and solid make-up techniques, you can still look good and feel great.

MAKE-UP

Your make-up routine will be established, but it is time to say goodbye to the colors you have been wearing for the past decades. It's most likely that your coloring is changing, often softening and cooling slightly.

KEY POINTS

- Defining your eyebrows is a must.

- Brown mascara is much more flattering than black.

- Concentrate your mascara on the outer edges of the eye, and do not apply to the lower lashes.

- The shape of your eyes may change, so consider different ways of applying your eye make-up to enhance them to their full potential (see pages 108–109).

- Use a good-quality foundation to even out skin tone.

- Powder only the bony parts of the face—forehead, nose, and chin—heavy powdering can tend to sit in fine lines and draw attention to them.

- If you are not powdering, use a cream blush, which can be more flattering.

- To give your mouth a fuller look, medium to light lipstick shades are more flattering than very dark browns and plums. A gloss in the center of the lips will help accentuate them.

COMMON PITFALLS

Some women at this age will consider undergoing invasive procedures such as Botox or surgery. However, there are ways of using your make-up to give your face a lift without the need for a surgeon's knife. If you feel that you are developing jowls or a double chin, a little darker powder or matte bronzer brushed along the jawline will help create the illusion of a firm face shape. Choose the correct foundation to avoid drawing attention to any lines, and go for natural shades for eyes and lips to suit your changing coloring.

SKINCARE ROUTINES FOR YOUR FIFTIES

Daily

- Cleanse and tone twice a day with gentle cleansers and skin fresheners.

- Use a skin serum underneath your moisturizer every day.

- Moisturize in the morning plus use an eye gel.

- Nourish with a rejuvenating night cream and eye cream before you go to bed.

Weekly

- Exfoliate only once a week.

- Use a firming, moisturizing mask once a week.

- Look for lotions and creams that contain vitamins C and E, which are antioxidants that protect against pollution and radiation, and are your best weapons against aging.

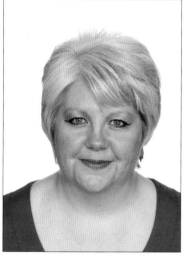

TRY TO AVOID…

Wearing the wrong colors of make-up for your coloring— getting the right colors at this age is more important than ever.

GET THE RIGHT LOOK

Fine lines will show up more with heavier foundations, so go for a light-textured foundation instead. Make sure that it still gives you enough coverage to hide any unevenness in skin tone. Use a lip pencil to define your lips and eyebrow pencil to define your eyebrows.

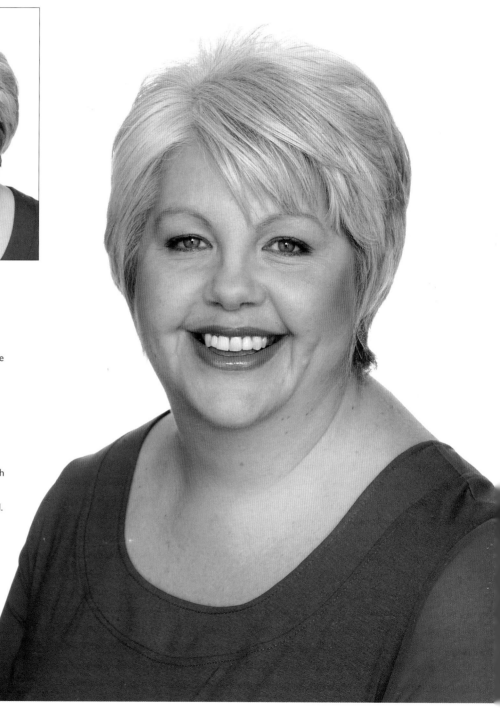

IN YOUR SIXTIES

Embrace the lines and furrows on your face as signs of a life well lived. This is not the time to give up on your make-up and skincare. On the contrary, your lifestyle may give you more opportunities for allowing yourself regular luxuries such as facials and other pampering treatments. Your make-up look is under-stated and sophisticated, with defined eyes and lips to light up your face.

MAKE-UP

Your skin will start to be noticeably thinner, so make-up application needs a light touch. It's a good idea to invest in a magnifying mirror to help you when putting on eye make-up without your glasses on.

KEY POINTS

- Smoothing skin primers will help give your skin an even texture before applying foundation.

- Liquid foundations are better than creamy ones, which tend to look heavy on the skin.

- Because the skin is finer, lighter concealers are preferable to heavier ones, which tend to sit on the skin.

- Shape your eyebrows regularly, then define with an eyebrow pencil to match your eyebrow color.

- Brown mascara is much more flattering than black.

- Avoid mascaras with lash builders, which can make the lashes appear clogged.

- Eye pencil used halfway under the eye creates the illusion of lifting the outer edge of the eye.

- Use blush to give definition and color.

- After applying lipstick and blotting, reapply lip pencil along the edge to prevent the color from bleeding.

COMMON PITFALLS

Avoid very shiny and/or frosted eye shadows, which cause creasing and also have a dated look. Avoid heavy powdering around the eye area, which will highlight any creases. Only use loose powder on the bony parts of your face—forehead, nose, cheekbones, and chin.

SKINCARE ROUTINES FOR YOUR SIXTIES

Daily

- Cleanse and tone twice a day with gentle cleansers and skin fresheners.

- Use a skin serum under your moisturizer every day.

- Moisturize the face and use an eye gel in the morning.

- Nourish with a rejuvenating night cream and eye cream before you go to bed.

Weekly

- Exfoliate only once a week.

- Use a firming, moisturizing mask once a week.

- Look for lotions and creams that contain vitamins C and E, which are antioxidants that protect against pollution and radiation, and are your best weapons against aging.

- Check for random facial hair, which tends to sprout around the upper lip and chin areas.

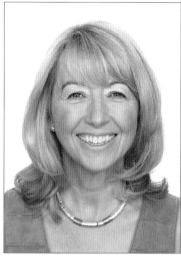

TRY TO AVOID…

Frosted and sparkly eye shadows, heavy eye liner, and light frosted lipsticks, which will give you a dated look.

GET THE RIGHT LOOK

Define your eyebrows gently with an eyebrow pencil that is close to your hair color. Go for liquid foundations, and powder only the bony parts of the face. Keep eye shadow colors matte and eye pencils to a medium depth. Define the lips with a lip pencil and avoid very dark colors if your lips are thin.

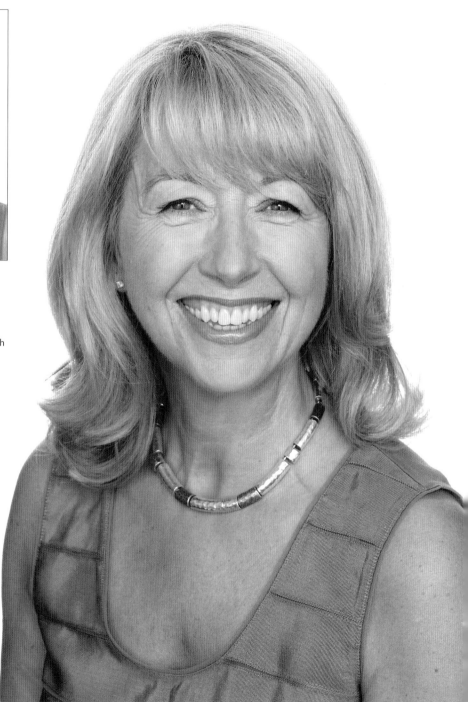

FLATTER
YOUR FACE

Make-up is not only a wonderful tool for bringing your face to life, it is also a fabulous, and pain-free, way to correct any of nature's imperfections—and enhance the good features with which you are blessed. Get to know your individual face shape, its proportions, and the characteristics of your facial features: eyes, nose, and lips. Use the following simple corrective make-up techniques and hairstyling tips to create your optimal look—to enhance your best features and disguise any areas you may wish to hide.

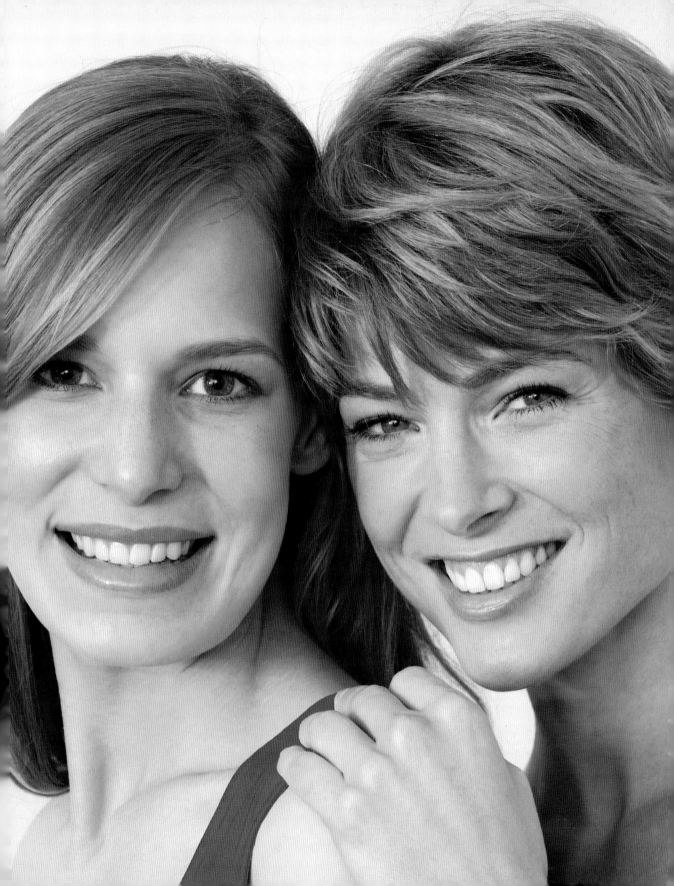

ENHANCE YOUR FACE

By using combinations of light and dark shading, you can create the illusion of having a perfectly formed oval face. First, you need to determine your face shape and proportions. To do so, sweep your hair back from your face and look straight into a mirror. See if your cheekbones are in line with the jaw and what is the width of your face in comparison with the length.

FACE SHAPE

The different face shapes require different corrective techniques to achieve an oval effect.

- **Oval:** An oval-shaped face will be wide at the cheekbones, gently sloping down to the jawline, with a gently rounded chin. The forehead will be slightly narrower than the cheekbones.

- **Square:** The cheekbones, forehead, and jaw will be in line with each other. The chin will be square onto the jawline and the width and the length of the face will be approximately the same.
  Corrective objective: To soften the jawline and highlight the cheekbones.

- **Rectangle:** The rectangle shape will have the cheekbones, forehead, and jaw in line with each other. The face will be longer than wider. Often, one proportion of the face—the forehead, the nose, or the lip to chin area—will be proportionally longer than the other areas.
  Corrective objective: To shorten the length of the face and also widen the width.

- **Inverted triangle:** An inverted triangle will have a wide forehead, narrowing at the cheekbones and to the jawline. The chin will often be pointed.
  Corrective objective: To narrow the forehead and give the jawline width.

- **Round:** A round face will have full cheeks, a rounded hairline, and rounded jawline and chin.
  Corrective objective: To take the fullness away from the sides of the face and to create the illusion of sharper cheekbones, forehead, and chin.

PROPORTIONS

A balanced face is one that is perfectly proportioned. The face can be divided into three sections, which should be equal in length: section 1 is from the hairline to the top of the bridge of the nose; section 2 is from the top of the bridge to the tip of the nose; section 3 is from the tip of the nose to the chin. All three sections will be the same length in a balanced face. By using a combination of corrective make-up and hairstyle techniques you can disguise any imbalance in shape and proportions.

CORRECTIVE TECHNIQUES

Using a combination of different shades of foundation, blushes, and highlighters, you can create the illusion of changing your face shape and features. Dark colors will minimize an area: try using a foundation one shade darker than you normally wear, or use bronzing powder. Light colors, such as highlighting eye shadows, light blushes, or iridescent highlighters, will enhance features. Always counterbalance shading with highlighting.

FACE SHAPE TIP

To help determine your face shape, take a lip or eye pencil and draw around your reflection on a mirror. This will give an outline to your face.

AN OVAL FACE

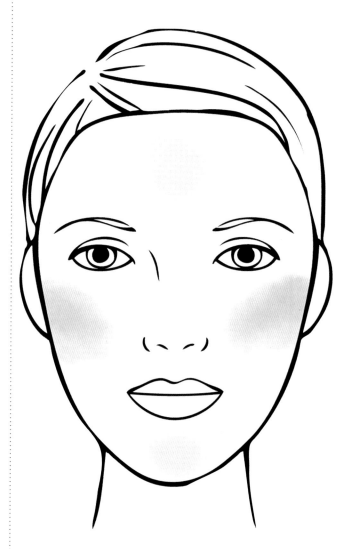

SHADING AND CONTOURING

You may not need to use a vast amount of corrective make-up, as you have a perfect face shape. Use blush to enhance your cheekbones and add a touch of iridescent highlighter on your forehead and chin. A whisk of blush along the forehead and the tip of your chin will give you a healthy glow.

HAIRSTYLES

Most hairstyles will complement your oval-shape face. Take into account the length of your neck and whether your ears stick out. Hair swept up, or even tucked behind the ears, will often enhance your striking bone structure.

GLASSES

When choosing your glasses, consider the length of your nose and whether you need to adjust the placement of the bridge. If you have a long nose, have a lower bridge and a shorter nose, or a high bridge, most styles will suit you, but avoid heavy-framed, masculine styles.

Blush

Highlighter

Shader

A SQUARE FACE

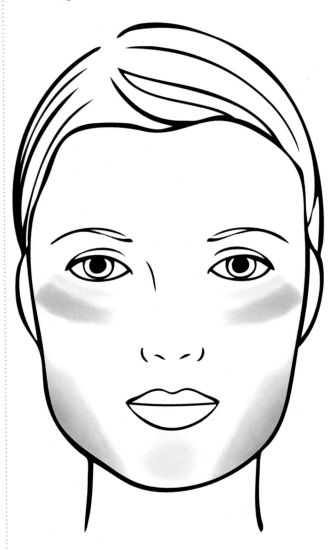

SHADING AND CONTOURING

To create the appearance of an oval-shaped face, you need to shade along the jawline with a slightly darker shade of foundation or bronzing powder. Then, apply iridescent highlighter along the top of the cheekbones, with your blush (slightly curved) directly underneath, to give the cheeks definition and draw the eye away from the shading.

HAIRSTYLES

You need to add volume and width to the temples with layering and some fullness. Hairstyles that taper to the chin are also flattering. Avoid heavy square bangs and straight bobs that finish at the jawline.

GLASSES

Look for frames that are oval or with rounded edges to soften the lines on your face. Avoid very square or rectangular frames, which will only emphasize the angles on your face.

Blush

Highlighter

Shader

A RECTANGULAR FACE

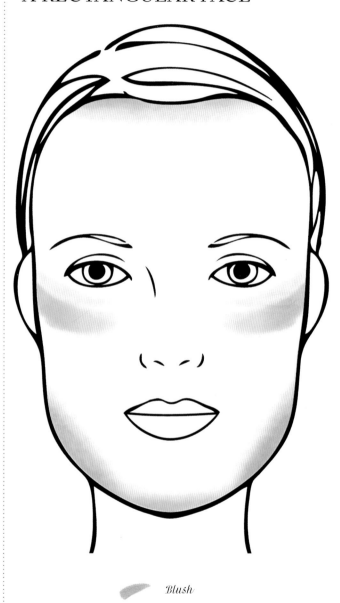

Blush

Highlighter

Shader

SHADING AND CONTOURING

To create the illusion of an oval-shaped face, you need to shorten the face and add width. Shade slightly under the tip of the chin and across the top of the forehead with a slightly darker foundation or bronzer and contour along the jawline. Next, add iridescent highlighter to the tops of the cheekbones, with blush applied directly below—this will give the illusion of added width. Try not to use blush too far down the cheeks, as this will give the appearance of hollow cheeks, making the face look longer. The eye area can be widened by adding length to the eyebrows with an eyebrow pencil and by slightly extending eye shadow and eye pencil to the outer edge of the eye.

HAIRSTYLES

This is probably the easiest way to balance a rectangular face. Bangs will shorten the face immediately. Adding width at the temples through layers or volume will also balance the face. Avoid center parts and long, straight hair, which will only elongate the look of the face.

GLASSES

The aim is to add width to the face, so look for oval, rimless, or semi-rimless frames. Go for wider arms that break up the length of the face and thus give the illusion of shortening it.

AN INVERTED TRIANGLE FACE

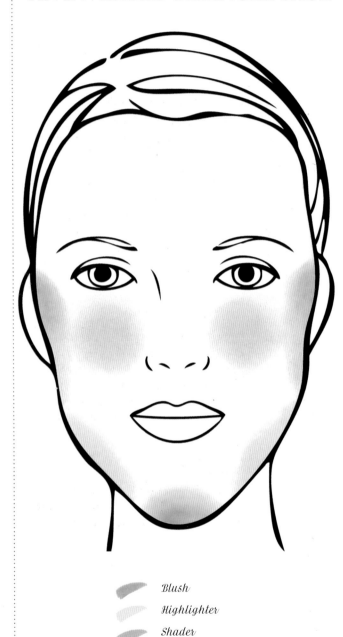

Blush

Highlighter

Shader

SHADING AND CONTOURING

To balance the face, use your slightly darker foundation/bronzer to shade the outer edges of the cheekbones and iridescent highlighter along the jawline. If you have a pointed chin, apply shading on the tip of the chin as well. Blush should be applied to the apples of the cheek. Be careful not to extend eye shadow beyond the outer edge of the eyes. Use the brightest lipstick or gloss from your palette, which will draw attention to the lower half of the face.

HAIRSTYLES

The principle here is to have a hairstyle that brings attention to the jawline. Long layers or flicked-out hairstyles that finish at the jawline work incredibly well. Hairstyles that come forward onto the cheekbones also help minimize the width of the face. Avoid styles where most of the volume is at the temple and there is no hair at the jawline.

GLASSES

A small, oval, or rounded shape will be best. Avoid wide, rectangular, or winged-up styles.

A ROUND FACE

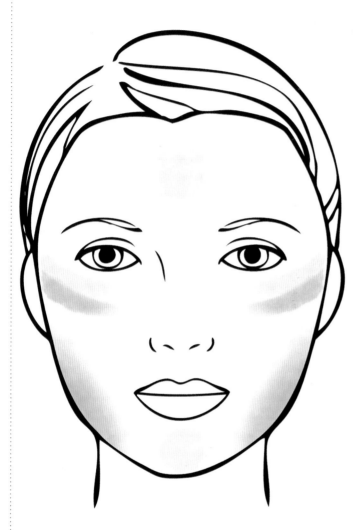

Blush

Highlighter

Shader

SHADING AND CONTOURING

Apply shading along the fullest part of your jawline. Highlight along the top of the cheeks, then apply your blush in a straight line below. Highlight the center of your forehead and chin with iridescent highlighter. Avoid applying your blush just on the apples of your cheeks. Eyebrows are best kept straight rather than arched. Apply eye shadows in straight lines, rather than rounded. Try to create a slightly wider and thinner mouth when lining your lips with lip pencil.

HAIRSTYLES

The aim is to create the illusion of an oval-shaped face. This can be achieved by soft layering coming forward onto the sides of the face. Straight or graduated bangs also help hide the rounded hairline. A straight bob will be balancing. Avoid full and rounded, curly hairstyles.

GLASSES

Any shape frame with angles, such as square or rectangular shapes, is perfect. Avoid full, rounded shapes, although flat oval shapes can work.

ENHANCE YOUR EYES

Your eyes say so much about yourself—make the most of them. Eye make-up can enhance the shape of any eye if used correctly and is one of the easiest ways to correct an unbalanced shape. Rather than just following make-up trends, it is important to understand the shape of your eye and how to make the most of it.

DIFFERENT EYE SHAPES

- **Proportioned eye:** The perfectly proportioned eye shape is the almond. When the eye is open you see one-third eyelid and two-thirds brow area. This shape can wear all different styles of eye make-up.
Corrective objective: Enhance rather than minimize.

- **Hooded eye:** A hooded eye is one where there is very little eyelid showing and the upper part of the lid folds over the lower eyelid.
Corrective objective: To create the illusion of a fuller lid, use light colors on the lid and contouring colors along the brow area.

- **Protruding eye:** A protruding eye is one where you see more eyelid, which seems to come forward. Generally there is very little brow area.
Corrective objective: To minimize the lid and make the brow area appear larger. Generous use of mascara helps minimize the protruding eyelid.

- **Deep-set eye:** The area surrounding this type of eye is often quite small. The eye appears to be set deep into the skull. Often very little eyelid can be seen.
Corrective objective: To make the whole eye area seem larger and come forward.

CORRECTIVE TECHNIQUES

The rule when applying make-up is simple: dark pencils and eye shadows minimize areas on the eye, whereas light and frosted/shimmer shades will highlight and enhance an area. A combination of different shades can help you change the appearance of the eye. Shaping your eyebrows is also important in enhancing your eyes. See page 110 for how best to define your eyebrows for your eye shape.

A PROPORTIONED EYE

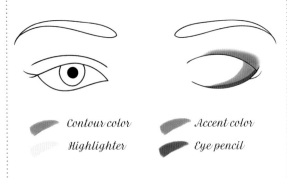

Contour color *Accent color*
Highlighter *Eye pencil*

ENHANCING THE SHAPE

Apply a highlighter shade over all the eye area. With an eye pencil, line the upper lash line by two-thirds and bottom lash line by one-third, both from the outer corner in. Then, add a contour color along two-thirds of the orbital bone. Add an accent color to the upper lid in a triangular shape in the outer corner of the eye. Finally, apply a blender shade to the center of the eyelid, using it to blend all the shades together.

A HOODED EYE

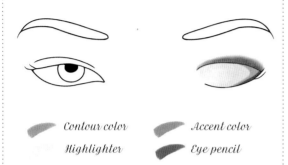

Contour color *Accent color*
Highlighter *Eye pencil*

CREATING A FULLER LID

Apply a highlighter shade all over the eye area. Use eye pencil along the top third of the lash line, from the outer corner inward and two-thirds on the bottom lash line. Apply a contour shade along the orbital bone. Add an accent color along the eye pencil, keeping it very thin, then apply the lightest blender color in your palette on the eyelid and lightly over the contour shade.

A PROTRUDING EYE

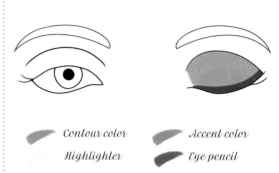

Contour color *Accent color*
Highlighter *Eye pencil*

MINIMIZING THE EYELID

Apply a highlighter shade all over the eye area. Using the darkest shade of eye pencil in your palette, apply a thick line along the top of the lash line all the way, then apply halfway along the bottom lash line. Next, apply the darkest shade of accent color over the eye liner and the rest of the eyelid. To finish, apply your blender color to blend all colors together.

A DEEP-SET EYE

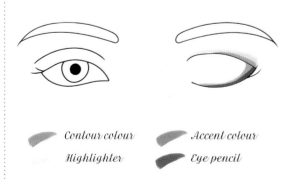

Contour colour *Accent colour*
Highlighter *Eye pencil*

ENLARGING THE EYE

Apply a highlighter shade all over the eye area. Use the brightest or lightest eye pencil from your palette to apply a thin line two-thirds along the top lash and one-third on the bottom. Add a light or bright accent color from the center of the orbital bone going outward onto the outer edge of the eye and then along the top and bottom lash lines. Use the lightest blender shade (frosted and shimmer eye shadows are ideal) directly in the eye socket.

ENHANCE YOUR EYEBROWS

Well-defined eyebrows are extremely flattering and add strength to your eyes. Some women notice that having a well-shaped brow can act as a non-surgical eye lift, too (see pages 116–117 for shaping tips). Making up your brows is a key make-up step, since its effect is so dramatic. You can achieve this with eyebrow pencils or powders and even some shades of eye shadows.

If you're simply enhancing the color of your natural brows, powders are best. However, to fill in gaps or reshape, pencils are more effective.

USING EYEBROW PENCILS

- For light or sparse eyebrows, fill in with a waxy eyebrow pencil in a natural color, like blonde.

- Brush the brows to remove any make-up.

- To enhance the color of the brows, only apply pencil to the hairs, not the skin.

- If you are drawing in to replace missing hairs, apply the pencil in short strokes, not one harsh line, so that the lines look like hair from a distance.

- Brush the eyebrows again to blend the pencil into the brow effectively—nothing looks more aging than a harsh, strong line.

USING EYE SHADOWS

- Use a small, hard, flat brush with an angled tip.

- Dip the brush into the powder, then tap on the edge of your hand to remove any loose particles.

- Starting at the widest edge of the brow, gently brush the shadow on using light, feathery, short strokes.

- If you need to lengthen your brows, apply the powder to the skin.

- If you have very dark eyebrows, you may find that using a dark brown eye shadow is more effective than pencils to fill in the brows.

MAKE-UP TIP
Use clear mascara to keep unruly eyebrows in place. Apply after you have filled in your brows.

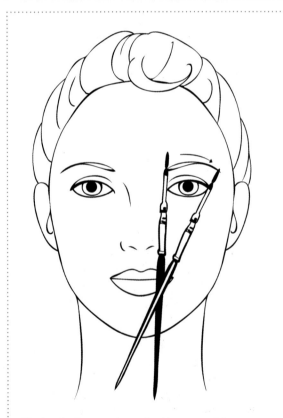

The length of your eyebrow should start parallel to the side of your nose and finish at the outer corner of the eye.

ENHANCE YOUR LIPS

Changing the appearance of your lips is easy to achieve with a combination of lip pencil, lipstick, and gloss. The mouth should be balanced, with the top and bottom lip even in size, and for a perfect length it should line up with your pupils. Choosing the right depth of color for your lipstick is important: lighter shades will give a fuller mouth and darker shades a smaller mouth.

THIN LIPS

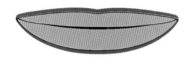

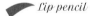 *Lip pencil*    *Lipstick*

Using the lightest lip pencil from your palette, draw a line on the outer edge of your lips, then fill in. Apply the lightest shade of lipstick all over, blot, and then apply lip gloss to the center of your lips. For extra fullness, a touch of iridescent highlighter on top of the cupid's bow will give the illusion of a fuller top lip.

UNEVEN LIPS

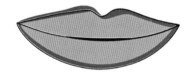

 Lip pencil    *Lipstick*

Depending on which lip is fuller, top or bottom, draw a line on the inside edge of the fuller lip and a line outside the natural lip line on the narrower lip with a lip pencil, and fill in. Apply a light lipstick to the smaller lip and a darker shade to the fuller lip: lightly press the lips to blend the colors. Only apply gloss to the narrower lip.

FULL LIPS

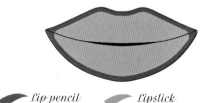

Lip pencil   *Lipstick*

When applying your foundation, take it over the lips, too. Then, using the darkest shade of lip pencil from your palette, draw the pencil inside the natural lip line and fill in. Apply lipstick just up to the edge of the lip pencil line. A matte cream lipstick is better for a full lip than a frosted one.

WIDE MOUTH

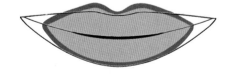

 Lip pencil    *Lipstick*

Using your lip pencil, draw a line outside the outer edge of the upper lip and inside the lower lip line and fill in. Don't extend into the corners of the mouth. Apply lipstick to the center of the mouth, then work outward applying less to the outer edges. Blot and apply lip gloss to the center of the top and bottom lips.

ENHANCE YOUR NOSE

Before taking extreme steps and considering plastic surgery to change the shape of your nose, you can create the illusion of changing its shape by using different shades of foundation and iridescent highlighters. If you are applying corrective make-up to change the shape of your nose, wear interesting eye make-up, a striking lipstick, or blush to draw attention elsewhere.

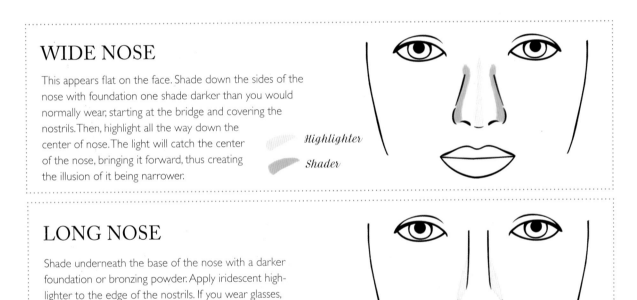

WIDE NOSE

This appears flat on the face. Shade down the sides of the nose with foundation one shade darker than you would normally wear, starting at the bridge and covering the nostrils. Then, highlight all the way down the center of nose. The light will catch the center of the nose, bringing it forward, thus creating the illusion of it being narrower.

Highlighter

Shader

LONG NOSE

Shade underneath the base of the nose with a darker foundation or bronzing powder. Apply iridescent highlighter to the edge of the nostrils. If you wear glasses, look for frames that have a low bridge.

Highlighter

Shader

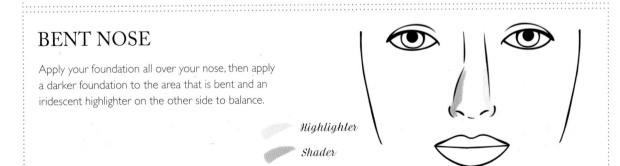

BENT NOSE

Apply your foundation all over your nose, then apply a darker foundation to the area that is bent and an iridescent highlighter on the other side to balance.

Highlighter

Shader

ENHANCE YOUR CHIN

If you are unhappy with the shape of your chin, you can use make-up to create the illusion of a shapely and balanced look to your face. It's not necessary to resort to chin or cheek implants. Some women lose the definition in their chin when they gain a little weight, and as we age, the facial muscles slacken. A little bronzer will do wonders for an instant lift.

POINTY CHIN

Apply a darker shade of foundation or shader to the prominent part of the chin, then apply an iridescent highlighter to the tip of the nose. Lastly, blend in with your normal foundation. Don't forget to apply a striking eye make-up and balance this with a neutral shade of lipstick.

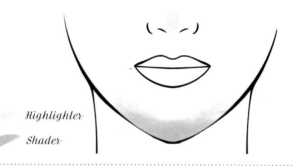

Highlighter

Shader

DOUBLE CHIN

The easiest way to disguise a double chin is by whisking bronzer along the jawline and under the chin and applying a little highlighter to the chin. See pages 24–25 for facial workout exercises that will help retain chin and neck shape.

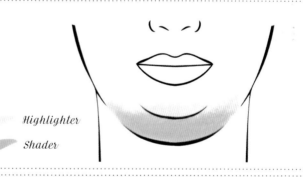

Highlighter

Shader

RECEDING CHIN

The aim is to make the chin appear more prominent, so apply an iridescent highlighter to the chin. Apply a darker shade of foundation or bronzer to the philtrum —the area between the top of the upper lip and the base of the nose. A bright lipstick will also help balance a receding chin.

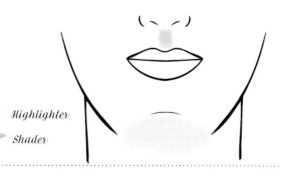

Highlighter

Shader

FINISHING TOUCHES

The final step to achieving your perfect look is to ensure that you are well turned out. It would be a shame to have great skin and perfect make-up, only for people to be distracted by messy eyebrows, poor dental hygiene, rough hands, and untidy hair. A beauty regime is something that needs to be kept up and should be habitual. You do not always need to consult a professional; most treatments can be easily done at home once you know how.

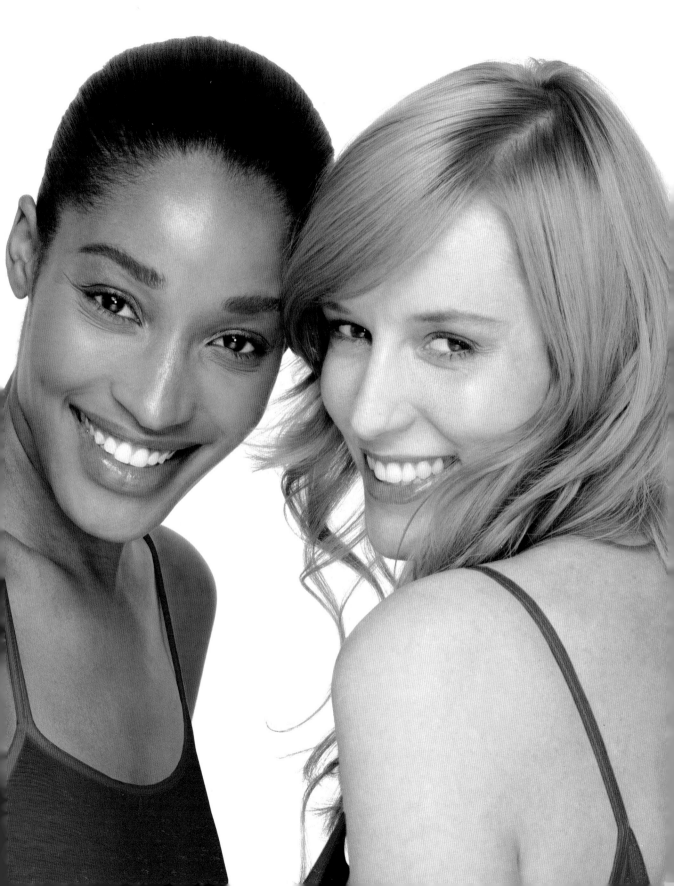

BROWS AND LASHES

Your eyebrows and lashes are like the mount and frame of a picture. They can make or break your whole make-up look, and for some people just grooming their eyebrows first thing in the morning gives them a made-up appearance. Similarly, your eyelashes add depth and interest to your eyes. Taking a little time to perfect their effect will be worth the effort.

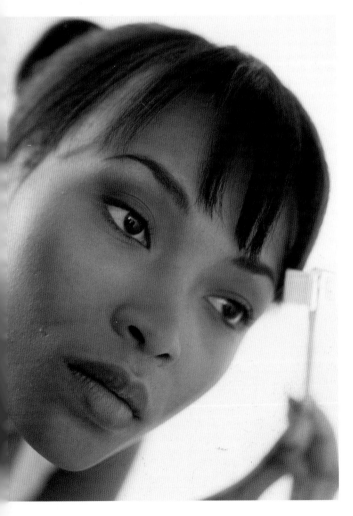

ABOVE **Using an eyebrow brush, brush your brows in the wrong direction to remove any make-up, and then brush back into place.**

EYEBROWS

Eyebrows can fade or may thin with age or because of overplucking. They can even change color and become a bit more unruly over time.

If you have never had your eyebrows shaped before or have unruly eyebrows, the first stage is to get them professionally shaped. This will give you a guideline for shaping them yourself. Ensure that you are prepared:

- Invest in a good pair of tweezers—a flat-ended pair is easier to use, as it has a tighter grip.
- If you have a low pain threshold, apply an ice cube along the eyebrow area to numb the skin.
- Good lighting is key when shaping, so that you can see all the hairs that need to be removed.

SHAPING YOUR EYEBROWS

The key to getting the right shape for your face is to find out where your brows should start, where they should end, and where they should arch.

If starting from scratch, use an eyebrow pencil to draw in your ideal eyebrow shape—this is especially helpful for blondes who have light eyebrows. Start by plucking all the hairs that fall outside that shape. Next, remove the hairs above the nose.

Remove a few stray hairs at a time on one eye, then move to the other eye to achieve a balanced look. Continue until the required shape is achieved. Wipe the brow frequently with a cotton pad soaked in toner to remove lose hairs. The following tips will help you achieve a good shape:

- The highest point of the arch in your eyebrow should line up with the outer edge of your iris. Tweeze out any hairs that fall under that arch.

- An arch to the eyebrow can give the illusion of an instant eye lift—just make sure it works with your face shape (see pages 102–107).

- To correct the shape of your eyebrow, it may be necessary for you to remove stragglers from above the eyebrow, but stragglers only—do not change the upper line of your eyebrows.

COLORING YOUR EYEBROWS

If your eyebrows are very light or have faded, consider having them professionally tinted. Tattooed eyebrows can be a very harsh look and are not advisable. See page 110 for using make-up to enhance the shape and color of your eyebrows.

EYELASHES

One of the most important aspects of having luscious lashes is to ensure that you remove mascara properly at the end of every day with a gentle eye make-up remover. Mascara contains adhesive, which will dry up the natural oils in your lashes and can make them brittle. Leaving your mascara on overnight will increase the risk of them breaking. Our lashes are constantly renewing themselves, and new lashes push up old ones. As we age, however, they can thin.

If your lashes tend to be very straight, try using an eyelash curler. This is placed at the base of the lashes and gently curves the lashes up.

TINTING YOUR EYELASHES

An instant lift to the lashes can be achieved by tinting: a must for someone with light coloring or if you are going on vacation and still want to look good without wearing make-up. Always have a skin test before you embark on tinting your brows or lashes to make sure that you are not allergic to the product.

FALSE EYELASHES

If you are after a more dramatic look, consider applying false eyelashes—either permanent or temporary. Permanent lashes are individually applied to the base of the lash and will last approximately one month, until your old lash grows out. Temporary lashes come in a strip and are applied with an adhesive along the lash line—either all along or just on the outer edge. These are good for an evening out or a special event and should be removed at the end of the day.

FINISHING TOUCH TIP

You may need to groom your eyebrows every few days, depending on your coloring.

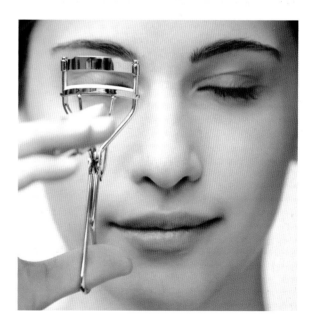

ABOVE **Curling your lashes is a great way to open up your eyes. Curlers can be applied before or after your mascara.**

CONTACT LENSES AND GLASSES

Glasses and contact lenses are often the finishing touch to a morning beauty routine, and there are a few special considerations to take into account when applying your make-up. In addition, consider your glasses frames as part of your make-up—their color and style are just as important as the make-up beneath, and this even applies to choosing sunglasses.

CONTACT LENSES

The main issue for contact lens wearers is to ensure that you avoid getting any products in your eye that will cause irritation with the lens. Some people prefer to apply their make-up with their lenses in, especially if they have a strong prescription. If so, remember:

- Cream eye shadows may be better than powder, which can irritate. If your favorite eye shadow is a powder, dampen the brush first to avoid fine particles of eye shadow getting on or under your lenses. Never line the inner eye with pencil or shadow.

- Waterproof mascara is a good choice for sensitive eyes, but avoid mascaras that contain fibers, which could irritate.

- When removing your make-up, remember to take your lenses out first, and avoid oily or greasy eye make-up remover, which may leave a film on your eye that will mist over your lenses.

- If you prefer to apply make-up with your lenses out, a magnifying mirror is essential.

GLASSES

The main thing to consider is the prescription of your glasses and what it does to the shape of your eye. Also consider the length of your lashes—sometimes applying a heavy mascara can cause your lashes to stroke the lenses of your glasses. Try tinting your lashes instead. Whatever your prescription, be sure to define your eyebrows with an eye pencil before you put your glasses on. Adjust your make-up to match your prescription:

IF YOU ARE NEARSIGHTED

- Avoid dark make-up colors, as these lenses can make eyes seem smaller.

- Always us natural or neutral tones and minimal eye pencils.

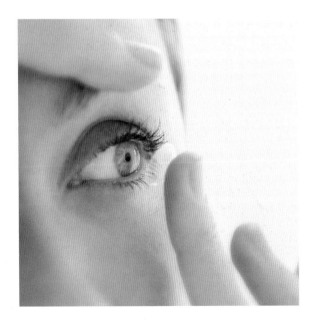

LEFT Remember to remove your contact lenses before taking off your eye make-up.

- Comb lashes and only apply a thin coating of mascara; curl your eyelashes to help them stand out.

- Pluck stray hairs in eyebrows.

IF YOU ARE LONG FARSIGHTED

- Aim to widen and deepen the eyes, as these lenses tend to make eyes come forward and magnify them.

- Eye pencils give eyes definition; use deeper shades of eye shadow to enhance eyes.

- Make sure your mascara doesn't clump on your lashes, which will make them look heavy.

CHOOSING GLASSES FRAMES

Your coloring (see pages 48–75) is an influential factor on getting your frames right. See also pages 102–107 for tips on matching frames to your face shape.

- **Light:** Choose light-colored frames, rimless or semi-rimless. Dark, heavy frames will completely distract from your face and are best avoided.

- **Deep:** Strong, dark-colored frames are best. If you have a small face and delicate features, make sure that the frame is lightweight but dark in color. Avoid rimless frames.

- **Warm:** The best shades of glasses need to have warmth to them, such as tortoiseshell, brown, gold, or amber. Rimless will work, but make sure that the arms and bridge of the nose have warm tones to them. When choosing sunglasses, opt for brown lenses as opposed to grey or black.

- **Cool:** The most flattering metallic frames for you will be silver and pewter. Frames in shades of blue, purple, and pink will also flatter your complexion. Sunglasses are best with blue-or grey-tinted lenses rather than brown or yellow.

- **Clear:** Brightly colored fashion shade frames are made for your coloring type. Whatever frame you choose, make sure the colour will work with most of the shades in your wardrobe. Check that the size

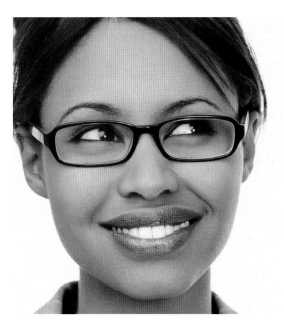

ABOVE **Consider your face shape, eye shape, and coloring when choosing the shape and color of frame for your glasses.**

of the frame doesn't overpower the size and scale of your face. Since your eyes are such a fabulous feature of your look, consider contact lenses as a great alternative to glasses.

- **Soft:** Metal frames are best if matte—either in gold, silver, pewter, or bronze. Tortoiseshell frames, rimless or semi-rimless, also work well.

FINISHING TOUCH TIPS

- For glasses and contact wearers, the first piece of equipment you need is a magnifying mirror; keep a large one in your bedroom or bathroom and a small handbag-size one to carry with you to help retouch your make-up during the day.

- Glasses may rub and remove your foundation; a dusting of powder after your foundation has been applied will help keep it in place.

HANDS AND FEET

Well-maintained hands and feet not only show that you care about your appearance but can make you feel good too—a flash of nail color is great for lifting your spirits. Uneven nails, chipped polish, and cracked heels will be distracting, even on a beautifully made-up person. Whether you go to a salon or do home treatments, give your hands and feet the attention they deserve.

HAND CARE

Hands generally show the signs of aging faster than the face, so it is important to pay special attention to them.

- **Moisturize:** Use a hand cream for moisturizing and protecting with SPF 15 or higher to prevent UV damage (see page 26). Research has found that age spots will actually fade somewhat if hands are no longer exposed to UV light. Always keep a jar of hand cream near the kitchen and bathroom sinks to apply after washing, and keep a nourishing cream by your bedside to apply at night before you go to sleep.

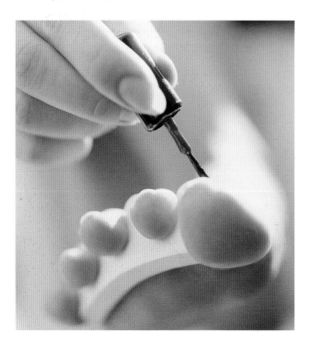

- **Protect:** Wear rubber gloves when doing any house-work that involves chemicals or when you are using your hands to do rough jobs such as gardening or home improvements. Wearing gloves in the winter months will also offer some protection against harsh winds and the cold, which can cause chapped skin.

- **Pamper:** A hand massage will stimulate the circulation and maintain flexibility. Even just rubbing the palm of your hand over the back of the other one as you wash them gives the skin on the surface of your hand some stimulation.

- **Exfoliate:** Use a hand exfoliating lotion at least once a week to keep your hands smooth. These will be coarser than ones used on your face.

FOOT CARE

It's easy to forget how hard working our feet are. We are on them all day, and they carry the total weight of our body. As women, we abuse them by forcing them into fashionable shoes with high heels or pointy toes and then wonder why we develop bunions and hard skin. There are several ways to take care of your feet.

- **Shoes:** Change the style of your shoes every day and vary the height of the heel. This will help keep your foot and calf muscles flexible. Going barefoot is also beneficial. If you are wearing sandals, don't forget

LEFT **Polished and shaped toenails are essential when wearing open-toe shoes or sandals.**

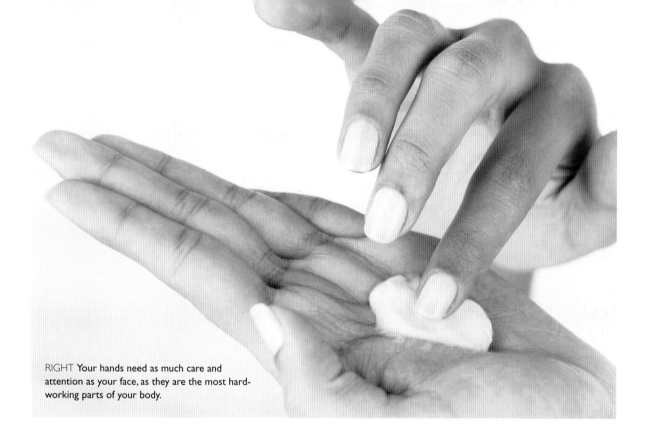

RIGHT **Your hands need as much care and attention as your face, as they are the most hard-working parts of your body.**

to apply a high-factor SPF cream to your feet in the morning, as your feet are exposed all day.

- **Soothe:** If you suffer from swollen ankles, try sitting with your feet raised above your heart for approximately 10 minutes, to reduce inflammation. Soaking your feet in a foot bath or roomy basin also helps soothe hot and tired feet.

- **Moisturize:** Daily treatment with an emery foot file after showering or bathing helps prevent a buildup of hard skin on your feet. Then, massage in rich foot cream to keep moisture in. If you suffer with particularly dry feet, apply your foot cream and put on socks before going to bed. The heat will help the cream be absorbed into the dry skin.

TOP TIPS FOR LOVELY NAILS

Manicured nails always make a good impression and are essential to a polished look. Healthy nails start with healthy nutrition—if your nails are brittle and break frequently, look at your diet to make sure you are getting the right vitamins and minerals (see pages 12–13).

- Avoid nail polish removers that contain acetone, which strips the nails of moisture.

- Gently push back cuticles after a bath or shower, when they will be softened, using your finger or a rubber hoof stick. If you have dry cuticles, massage in cuticle oil as well.

- Scrubbing nails with a fine nail brush will stimulate healthy growth from the nail bed and keep nails clean.

- Buff your nails regularly, as this also stimulates the circulation and helps prevent flaking.

- Always apply a base coat before applying colored nail polish. It provides a surface for the nail polish to stick to and stops your nails from becoming yellow over time.

- To make sure your manicure lasts, apply a top coat.

- Long-term use of false nails can cause damage—try to avoid if possible or only use for special occasions.

- Careful trimming of toenails is important to prevent ingrown nails. If they occur, seek advice from a chiropodist.

A WINNING SMILE

A perfect smile with gleaming teeth is one of the most attractive assets a woman can have. Taking care of your teeth on a regular basis will not only pay dividends in the short term but lengthen the life of your smile. Establish an oral healthcare routine, if you haven't already, and remember that regular trips to the dentist will keep your smile bright and your mouth healthy.

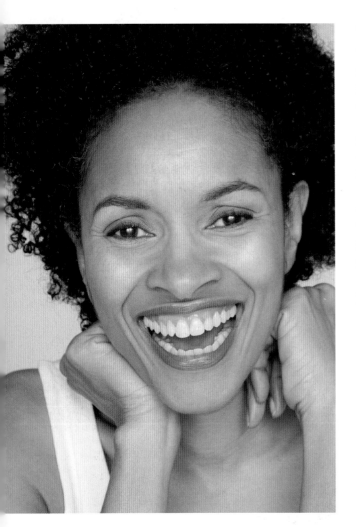

ABOVE **Dental hygiene is important for your overall well-being and health. No amount of make-up can hide an unsightly smile.**

TAKING CARE OF YOUR TEETH

The rules you learned as a child haven't changed: carefully brush your teeth twice a day and floss daily to remove plaque, which can lead to gum disease. Poor dental hygiene can also lead to bad breath, or halitosis.

If you wear dentures you still need to maintain regular oral healthcare, keeping them clean to prevent staining, bad breath, or gum irritation.

Consult your dentist or hygienist at least twice a year for a professional cleaning and oral examination, and remember to eat well—nutritional deficiency can cause gum disease, which can lead to tooth loss.

PROFESSIONAL TREATMENTS

- **Scaling and polishing** is normally done every six months by a hygienist to remove the buildup of plaque.
- **Bleaching** is becoming increasingly popular and should only be done professionally by your dentist. A mold is made of your teeth, which is filled with a diluted solution to whiten the teeth.
- **Veneer** is a fine layer of porcelain that is bonded to the tooth permanently (although it can chip). This is used to reshape and recolor any problem teeth.
- **Crowns** The damaged tooth is shaped down to a peg and a replica is fitted over the top. Porcelain crowns are now increasingly used and last up to 20 years or more.

HAIR

A woman's hair is her crowning glory. Understanding your hair and how its style can enhance your face will save hours of anguish in front of the mirror. The most important aspect of hair care is finding the right hairdresser, who will not only make you look fabulous but also advise you on the best products for your hair type and style.

STYLING TIPS

When considering a new hairstyle, take into account your face shape (see pages 102–107) and also your lifestyle—if you have little time, choose a style that you can wash and go. If you are coloring your hair, choose a shade that works with your natural coloring. A good guide is the shade of your eyebrows.

Take care of your hair—to limit heat damage from a drier, wait until your hair is almost dry before you blow dry. At the end of drying, give your hair a blast of cold air, which will help make the styling last longer.

FINE HAIR

- **Style:** Layering is key to adding volume.
- **Volume:** Sometimes you can tease or backcomb to add volume, but it must be brushed out so as not to damage the hair shaft. A lightweight perm can also give volume and root lift.
- **Body:** Use a volumizing shampoo and a lightweight mousse when drying, and try drying your hair upside down, which will give root lift.

NATURALLY CURLY OR FRIZZY HAIR

- **Straighten:** Straighteners are great for a temporary look, but must be used on hair that is in good condition—the heat can dry and damage the hair shaft.
- **Smooth:** Before blow drying, apply a serum to control frizz. There are now professional treatments

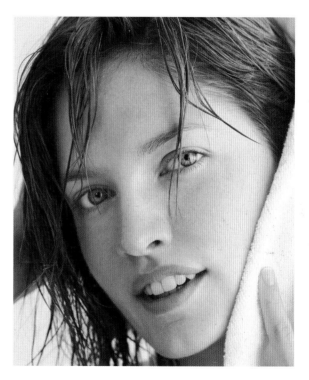

ABOVE Try to wait until your hair is almost dry before you start styling with a blow drier.

that smooth the outer cuticle of the hair shaft, making the hair straighter, softer and less frizzy.

THICK HAIR

- **Style:** Graduated layers will minimize the volume.
- **Smooth:** Use smoothing conditioners.

INDEX

ACKNOWLEDGMENTS

This is *the* book we've been wanting to do forever! We are both so passionate about make-up because we know first-hand how make-up can make you instantly feel confident and able to face the world, whatever it throws at you.

From our stable of Colour Me Beautiful consultants and glamorous models, we thank Kerry Ellis, Kathy Ennis, Anita Feron Clark, Angi Jones, Mandy Lehto, and Sharon Whittock for their time and charm in front of the camera.

Behind the scenes, we are truly appreciative of the beautiful work Victoria Barnes created when doing hair and make-up —exclusively using Colour Me Beautiful make-up—while Ruth Jenkinson, our incredible photographer, inspired us all and made it come alive.

Thanks to Jane Brown for her insightful knowledge of beauty therapy and to our husbands, Jim Henshaw for being our technical whiz and Peter Sirian for imparting his medical knowledge to the science parts of the book.

Huge thanks go to Stephanie Jackson for commissioning this book. The Hamlyn team has been a joy to work with yet again: Yasia Williams's fantastic design flare and Clare Churly's patience in guiding us through a new form of editorial process has really made this a book we are so proud of.

All the while we appreciated Veronique Henderson's beady eyes hovering reassuringly and for giving us the opportunity to write this book.

Finally, this has been a truly joint effort; we are proud to have been able to work together and with such a dedicated team of professionals.

Pat Henshaw and Audrey Hanna

PICTURE ACKNOWLEDGMENTS

All photographs are by Ruth Jenkinson for Octopus Publishing with the exception of the following:

Alamy Allstar Picture Library 57 right; Fancy 18; Form Advertising 119; I love images 21; Ian Hooton/Science Photo Library 13, 19; Image Source 115; MBI 12; Oleksiy Maksymenko Photography 10; Tom Merton 26. **Getty Images** Amana Productions 121; Astrid Stawiarz 61 right; Dave Hogan 69 left; David Cheskin 69 right; Eye Candy Images 9; François Durand 73 right; Frazer Harrison 61 center; Fuse 14; John Shearer/WireImage 65 left; Jon Feingersh 122; Julien M Hekimian 57 left; Karen Moskowitz 15; Kei Uesugi 16; Kevin Mazur/WireImage 53 left; Kevin Winter 73 center; Martin Poole 120; Matthew Wakem 23; Pando Hall/Photographers Choice 101; Steve Granitz/WireImage 53 right, 57 center; Thomas Northcut 27. **Image State** Royalty Free 17. **Photolibrary** Florian Franke/Superstock 116; Julian Winslow/Ableimages 117; V Beranger/Self Photos Agency 20. **Press Association Images** 73 left; Doug Peters/EMPICS Entertainment 65 center; Sipa Press 69 center. **Rex Features** Sipa Press 61 left, 65 right, 69 center; Startraks Photo 53 center.

Publishing Director: Stephanie Jackson
Managing Editor: Clare Churly
Deputy Art Director: Yasia Williams-Leedham
Picture Library Manager: Jennifer Veall
Photographer: Ruth Jenkinson
Hair and Make-up Artist: Victoria Barnes
Illustrator: Brogan Kingsley
Senior Production Controller: Caroline Alberti